Male Infertility
Problems and Perspectives

Male Infertility
Problems and Perspectives

Editor

Hemant Deshpande

Professor and Head
Department of Obstetrics and Gynecology
Dr DY Patil Medical College,
Dr DY Patil Vidhyapeeth DPU
Pimpri, Pune, Maharashtra

Co-Editor

Munjal Pandya

Assistant Professor
AMC MET Medical College
Sheth LG Hospital
Ahmedabad, Gujarat

Forewords

Shirish N Daftary
Dipti M Shah
Mukul Shah

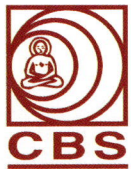

CBS

CBS Publishers & Distributors Pvt Ltd

New Delhi • Bengaluru • Chennai • Kochi • Kolkata • Mumbai
Bhopal • Bhubaneswar • Hyderabad • Jharkhand • Nagpur • Patna • Pune • Uttarakhand • Dhaka (Bangladesh)

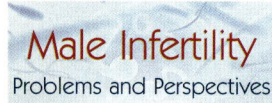

Male Infertility
Problems and Perspectives

ISBN: 978-93-88725-68-2

First Edition: 2019

Published by Satish Kumar Jain and produced by Varun Jain for

CBS Publishers & Distributors Pvt Ltd

4819/XI Prahlad Street, 24 Ansari Road, Daryaganj, New Delhi 110 002, India.
Ph: 23289259, 23266861, 23266867 Website: www.cbspd.com
Fax: 011-23243014   e-mail: delhi@cbspd.com; cbspubs@airtelmail.in.

Corporate Office: 204 FIE, Industrial Area, Patparganj, Delhi 110 092
Ph: 4934 4934   Fax: 4934 4935   e-mail: publishing@cbspd.com; publicity@cbspd.com

Branches

- **Bengaluru:** Seema House 2975, 17th Cross, K.R. Road, Banasankari 2nd Stage, Bengaluru 560 070, Karnataka
  Ph: +91-80-26771678/79   Fax: +91-80-26771680   e-mail: bangalore@cbspd.com
- **Chennai:** 7, Subbaraya Street, Shenoy Nagar, Chennai 600 030, Tamil Nadu
  Ph: +91-44-26680620/26681266   Fax: +91-44-42032115   e-mail: chennai@cbspd.com
- **Kochi:** 42/1325, 1326, Power House Road, Opp KSEB, Power House, Ernakulam 682 018, Kochi, Kerala
  Ph: +91-484-4059061-65   Fax: +91-484-4059065   e-mail: kochi@cbspd.com
- **Kolkata:** 6/B, Ground Floor, Rameswar Shaw Road, Kolkata-700 014, West Bengal
  Ph: +91-33-22891126, 22891127, 22891128   e-mail: kolkata@cbspd.com
- **Mumbai:** 83-C, Dr E Moses Road, Worli, Mumbai-400018, Maharashtra
  Ph: +91-22-24902340/41   Fax: +91-22-24902342   e-mail: mumbai@cbspd.com

Representatives

• **Bhopal** 0-8319310552	• **Bhubaneswar** 0-9911037372	• **Hyderabad** 0-9885175004	• **Jharkhand** 0-9811541605
• **Nagpur** 0-9421945513	• **Patna** 0-9334159340	• **Pune** 0-9623451994	• **Uttarakhand** 0-9716462459
• **Dhaka (Bangladesh)** 01912-003485			

Printed at: HT Media Ltd., Greater Noida, UP, India

to
Sadguru Raghvendra Swamiji

Contributors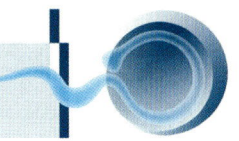

Ashok Kumar
Director, Professor
Department of Obstetrics and Gynaecology
Maulana Azad Medical College and
Lok Nayak Hospital, New Delhi, India
Chapter 1: Male Fertility: Global Scenario

Divya KV
Resident
Department of Obstetrics and Gynaecology
Maulana Azad Medical College and
Lok Nayak Hospital, New Delhi, India
Chapter 1: Male Fertility: Global Scenario

Yuvraj Jadeja
Assistant Professor
Department of Obstetrics and Gynaecology
Pramukhswami Medical College
Karamsad, Gujarat, India
Chapter 2: Male Factor Infertility

Nitin Raithatha
Professor
Department of Obstetrics and Gynaecology
Pramukhswami Medical College
Karamsad, Gujarat, India
Chapter 2: Male Factor Infertility

Atul Munshi
Ex-Professor and Head
Department of Obstetrics and Gynaecology
GCS Medical College
Ahmedabad, Gujarat, India
Chapter 3: Exercise, Lifestyle and Nutrition Role in Male Infertility

Amit Kharat
Professor
Department of Radiodiagnosis
Dr DY Patil Medical College
Pune, Maharashtra, India
Chapter 4: Imaging Modalities in Male Infertility

Nikith Somani MBBS
Resident
Department of Radiology
Dr DY Patil Medical College
Pune, Maharashtra, India
Chapter 4: Imaging Modalities in Male Infertility

Jacob Jason MBBS
Resident
Department of Radiology
Dr DY Patil Medical College
Pune, Maharashtra, India
Chapter 4: Imaging Modalities in Male Infertility

Charusheela R Gore
Professor
Department of Pathology
Dr DY Patil Medical College and Hospital
Pune, Maharashtra, India
Chapter 5: Semen Analysis

Anjali H Deshpande
Pathologist
Department of Pathology
Dr DY Patil Medical College and Hospital
Pune, Maharashtra, India
Chapter 5: Semen Analysis

Munjal Pandya MS (ObGyn)
Assistant Professor
Department of Obstetrics and Gynaecology
AMC MET Medical College and
Sheth LG Hospital
Ahmedabad, Gujarat, India
Chapter 5: Semen Analysis

Anand K Shinde MD (ObGyn)
Director Andrology and IVF Consultant
Deenanath Mangeshkar Superspeciality Hospital
Pune, Maharashtra, India
Chapter 6: Medical Management of Male Infertility

Shahaji Chavan
Professor and Head
Department of Surgery
Dr DY Patil Medical College
Pune, Maharashtra, India
Chapter 7: Surgical Management of Male Infertility

Yogendra Modi MS
Superintendent
SCL Municipal Hospital and
Smt. NHL Municipal Medical College
Ahmedabad, Gujarat, India
Chapter 7: Surgical Management of Male Infertility

Shrenik Shah (Urosurgeon)
Professor and Head
Department of Urology
BJ Medical College and Civil Hospital
Ahmedabad, Gujarat, India
Chapter 7: Surgical Management of Male Infertility

Manish Banker
Medical Director
Nova IVI Fertility
Ahmedabad, Gujarat, India
Past President
Indian Society for Assisted Reproduction (ISAR)
Chapter 8: IUI: Prerequisites, Counseling and Informed Consent

Neha Sharma
Fellow Reproductive Medicine
Nova IVI Fertility
Ahmedabad, Gujarat, India
Chapter 8: IUI: Prerequisites, Counseling and Informed Consent

Surykant Hayatnagarkar
Practising Pathologist
Director
Cryocell India Pvt. Ltd.
New Delhi, India
Chapter 9: Sperm Preparation Methods and Techniques of IUI

Hrishikesh D Pai MD FCPS FICOG MSc (USA)
Medical Director, Bloom IVF (Mumbai, Navi Mumbai, Delhi, Gurgaon, Mohali and Bengaluru)
Administrator
FOGSI Manyata Program
Director
International Affairs, International Federation of Fertility Societies
Adjunct Assistant Professor
Eastern Virginia Medical School USA
Postgraduate Teacher
DNB Gynecology Lilavati Hospital
Mumbai, India
Chapter 10: Factors Influencing Success of IUI

Manisha Kundnani MD FNB
Fertility Consultant, Fertility Square
The IVF Clinic
Mumbai, Maharashtra, India
Chapter 10: Factors Influencing Success of IUI

Nandita Palshetkar MD FCPS FICOG
Medical Director, Bloom IVF (Mumbai, Navi Mumbai, Delhi, Gurgaon, Mohali and Bengaluru)
Institutional Attachments:
President Elect, Federation of Obstetrics and Gynaecological Societies of India
Vice President, Indian Society for Assisted Reproduction
Chairperson, Maharashtra Chapter of ISAR
Chapter 10: Factors Influencing Success of IUI

Rishma Dhillon Pai MD DNB FRCOG FICOG FCPS DGO
Consultant Gynaecologist, Bloom IVF, Lilavati, Jaslok and Hinduja Healthcare Hospitals
Institutional Attachments:
President, Indian Society for Assisted Reproduction
President, Indian Association of Gynaecological Endoscopists
Imm. Past President, Federation of Obstetric and Gynaecological Societies of India
Chapter 10: Factors Influencing Success of IUI

Rohan Palshetkar MS
Gynaecologist
Dr. DY Patil Medical College, Hospital and Research Centre
Mumbai, Maharashtra, India
Institutional Attachments:
Member, Youth Council MOGS
Mumbai, Maharashtra, India
Chapter 10: Factors Influencing Success of IUI

Anjali Malpani MD
Malpani Infertility Clinic
Colaba, Mumbai, India
Chapter 11: Sperm Banking: A Solution to all Problems

Aniruddha Malpani MD
Malpani Infertility Clinic
Colaba, Mumbai, India
Chapter 11: Sperm Banking: A Solution to all Problems

Manish Machave MD DNB MNAMS LLB Dip Endoscopy (Germany), Adv Dip Gyn Endoscopy (France)
Unit Head and PG Teacher
Kamla Nehru Hospital
National Coordinator
FOGSI Ethics and Medicolegal Committee
Chapter 12: Medicolegal Aspect of IUI

Foreword

Procreation is a basic human instinct and a natural consequence of marriage. Family constitutes the basic unit of society on which it thrives. Inability to procreate is looked upon with disdain. For long it was considered that if a man could consummate his marriage, then the cause of inability to bear a child was attributed entirely to his wife. Such a couple suffered from social stigma and was often ostracised.

The Times of India (2017) reported that India bears a large burden of infertility. They reported an estimated burden of 22–33 million infertile couples in the country and further reported the incidence to be rising. Late age of marriage, career considerations, contraceptive use for long, lifestyle changes, work stress, poor nutrition and indulgence in tobacco, alcohol and drugs have added to this problem. Genital tuberculosis and high prevalence of sexually transmitted diseases have taken a toll too.

The incidence of infertility in India is estimated to be between 10 and 15%, WHO estimated the incidence of infertility to vary widely in India, being lowest in Uttar Pradesh (3.7%) to being highest in Kashmir (15%). Infertility rates appear to be rising at an alarming rate in urban areas.

Male factor is estimated to contribute towards infertility in 30–40% of cases. The reluctance on the part of the male partner to subject himself to medical check-up has gradually yielded to cooperation. Modern techniques of investigation and treatment has brought hope and reward in the lives of many couples who had resigned themselves to a life of ignominy.

My compliments to Prof (Dr) Hemant Deshpande and his team for bringing together so many experts to contribute chapters to this manual. The concise information provided will be immensely useful to the practitioner to adopt modern day therapeutic advances to treat patients under their care.

I wish this book a resounding success.

Dr Shirish N Daftary MD DGO FICOG
Prof Emeritus, Obstetrics and Gynaecology
Nowrosjee Wadia Maternity Hospital, Mumbai

Ex-Dean and Medical Advisor
Nowrosjee Wadia Maternity Hospital. Mumbai

Ex-Joint Associate Editor
Journal of Obstetrics and Gynaecology of India

Past President
Bombay Obstetric and Gynaec. Society

Past President
FOGSI

Editor
Shaw's Textbook of Gynaecology, Holland and Brews
Manual of obstetrics, Arias—High Risk Pregnancy and many other publications

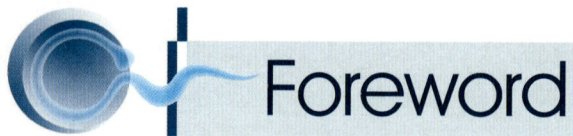

Foreword

This book, *Male infertility: Problems and Perspectives* focuses on various aspects of male infertility with their solutions. Nowadays with advancement of artificial reproductive technologies, it has become possible for the couple to conceive even in difficult cases of infertility, but then, getting into the root of the cause/causes of infertility still remains the step of utmost importance.

My best wishes are with Dr Hemant Deshpande and his team of experts, for their efforts of spreading basic as well as updated knowledge throughout the society.

Dr Dipti M Shah
Dean, Professor. Obstetrics and Gynaecology
AMC MET Medical College
Sheth LG Hospital

Ex-Deputy Mayor
Ahmedabad Municipal Corporation, Ahmedabad

Foreword

An infertile couple most of the times carries the burden of social pressure. This work of Dr Hemant Deshpande and his team will enlighten the readers with its exclusive focus on male infertility, with its causes, investigations and treatment with recent updates.

It is an addition to a long list of such helpful academic literatures by my dear friend Dr Deshpande.

I once again congratulate him and the team for their efforts and my best wishes.

Dr Mukul Shah
Professor. Obstetrics and Gynaecology
GCS Medical College

Ex-Deputy Mayor
Ahmedabad Municipal Corporation, Ahmedabad

Preface

This book titled *Male Infertility: Problems and Perspectives* reflects contemporary opinions of infertility experts and andrologists in the domain of male infertility.

Sir William Osler, the father of modern medicine, had rightly stated that the two basic drives of mankind are *To get and to beget*.

For ages the widely prevalent belief in society was that if the man could consummate the marriage, then the fault of inability to beget an offspring lay squarely with the wife. This belief was so widely prevalent in society that since times immemorial, women who could not bear a child, have been castigated and condemned to a life of ignominy.

Advances in science coupled with studies and research carried on over the last few decades have amply proven the culpability of the male, who plays a significant role in the highly complex issue of infertility. Studies have revealed many factors contributing to male subfertility. These have been identified and treatment modalities too have evolved to treat these effectively. The drive for procreation is extremely strong and has employed technology to design diagnostic tests and treatment protocols to address the scourge of barrenness.

The revolution in the field of *Male Infertility*, the rich, varied experience of Indian infertility experts collaborating with andrologists motivated us to invite specialists to share their expertise and experiences. They have made this possible by contributing their invaluable inputs to this publication.

The last few decades have witnessed a paradigm shift to the profile of couples seeking medical assistance to combat infertility. Couples often are inclined to differ having babies to a later age. Pressures of education, career compulsions and longer periods of using contraceptives has led to delay in child bearing. The advancing age becomes a crucial factor rendering the couple more vulnerable to an *age related decrease in fecundity*.

The mother is in her middle age when she starts her family. Modern day couples are marrying late and postponing childbearing. The *Sexual Revolution* has provided this generation with an unprecedented control over fertility. A consequence of this behaviour pattern has been a rise in the incidence of STDs, repeated abortions—often induced, and prolonged exposure to occupational and environmental hazards.

Important aspects of male infertility have been discussed by experts, they have shared their experiences with colleagues to help them provide high quality care to their patients. This book will certainly be a boon, both to the medical fraternity as well as the erudite generation to understand and deal with this highly essential and yet complex subject of infertility.

Hemant Deshpande
Munjal Pandya

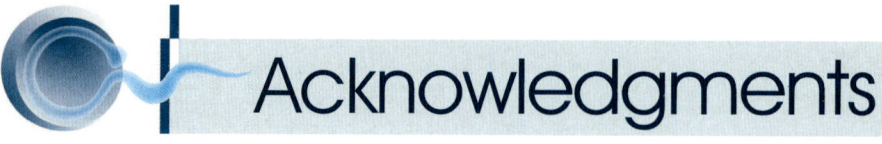

Acknowledgments

This book covers multiple facets of fertility problems with focus on male issues and their respective solutions. The progress of technology has made us capable to solve many problems which were previously not manageable. The horizons have expanded with in-depth exploration of various causes, thus making the search for solution possible. This compilation of expert input from well-experienced and esteemed authors, cover all the basic aspects with the most recent updates. We hope this book helps readers to deliver optimal service to the society, so as to bring joy in the incomplete lives of infertile couples.

I would like to thank all my contributors for neatly and timely submission of articles for this book.

I would like to thank my wife Dr Anjali Deshpande for bearing with me and giving her time in making this book.

I will put on record my appreciation for Mr Ramesh Krishnamachari, Mr YN Arjuna and Ms Ritu Chawla of CBS Publishers & Distributors Pvt Ltd for assisting in the editorial process efficiently and promptly.

Hemant Deshpande

Contents

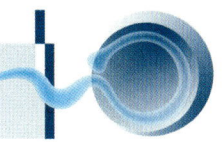

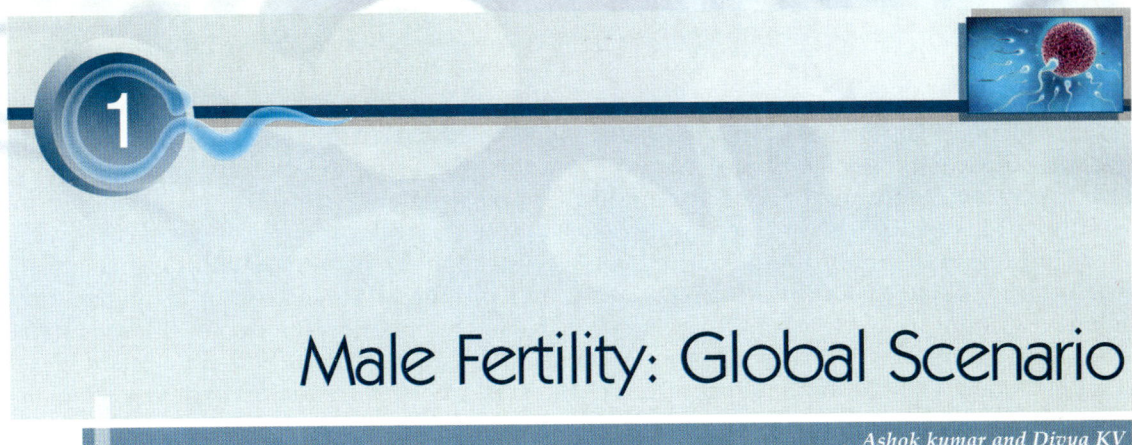

Male Fertility: Global Scenario

Ashok kumar and Divya KV

Infertility and subfertility have an effect on a major proportion of human population. Infertility is outlined as inability to conceive after one year of unprotected intercourse. Prevalence values of sterility is found to be 2.5 times larger among women as calculated by two year time frame. The burden in men is unknown. The burden of infertility/subfertility is generally underestimated and has displayed increasing trend over the last twenty years. The requirements of those couple who are unable to attain and maintain a desired pregnancy are not self-addressed, particularly in lower resource settings worldwide.[1]

World sterility prevalence rates are tough to work out, because of the presence of both male and feminine factors that complicate the estimation by solely addressing the female factors as an outcome of a pregnancy or nascency. One in each four couples in developing countries had been found to be littered with sterility, as found by responses from women on demographic survey. The burden remains high. A WHO analysis of demographic and health surveys knowledge 2004, calculable that over 186 million ever married women of procreative age in developing countries were maintaining a child wish, translating into one in each four couples.[1] Fertility issues have affected increasing range of couples in last decades and fertility rate in men under age of thirty years

has also been remittent worldwide by 15%.[2] Approximately 40% of sterility cases were involving men, 40% of women and 20% of both sexes.[3]

Mascarenhas et al found that 1.9% of women aged 20–44 years who wished to have children and were unable to own their initial nascency (primary infertility) and 10.5% of women with a previous nascency were unable to own an extra nascency (secondary infertility).[4] The prevalence of primary sterility was higher among girls aged 20–24 years than among older girls. The prevalence of primary sterility was 1.5% in America to a 2.6% in North Africa and also the Middle East. In India, the calculable prevalence of sterility is 12.6%–14.2%.[5,6] The reproductive anomalies or disorders in the male accounts for 50% of sterility and no detectable cause is found on routine tests in about 25% sterility cases in India.[7] The social burden of sterility in terms of branding, discrimination and ostracism falls on women who do not have children, though the underlying cause lies in their male partners.

Males with spermatozoa parameters below the WHO normal values are thought to have sterility.[8] The key abnormalities are low spermatozoan concentration (oligospermia), poor spermatozoan motility (asthenospermia), and abnormal spermatozoan morphology (teratospermia). Others abnormalities of volume and different seminal markers of epididymal, prostatic, and seminal vesicle function.[9] The burden of fertility issues is increasing over the globe in the recent years. The foremost common reasons for male infertility/subfertility are hormonal imbalances or blockages within the male procreative organs. Obstructions within the vas deferens account for up to twenty percent of male cases of infertility. Physical problems such as injuries to the male reproductive gland, radiation therapy, failure of sex gland descent and varicocoele are contributive factors for male fertility problems. Diabetes will cause erectile dysfunction because of reduced blood flow secondary to vascular damage. Thyrotoxicosis will have an effect on spermatozoon count and quality. Secretory abnormalities like low androgenic hormone level and infectious diseases like epididymitis, prostatitis or sexually transmitted diseases have impact on spermatozoon production. Testicular trauma and torsion are risk factors for male sterility. Precocious pubescence or delayed pubescence, exposure to harmful substances like lead, asbestos, cadmium, mercury, alkene chemical compound, exposure to high body temperatures as in staff close to furnaces, surgical injury to vas particularly following bilateral hernia repair are other causes for male infertility. Chronic renal and chronic liver disorders do have an association with male infertility.[10]

Occupational hazards are a crucial contributing factor for infertility. There is associated degree of proof regarding decline in sperm quality in recent years. The biological credibleness for a control of mobile phones on spermatozoon quality has to be thought of. Nonparticulate radiation discharged from mobile phones could have thermal and non-thermal effects on biological tissues. Nonthermal interactions are believed to extend the assembly of reactive oxygen species and this could cause DNA damage. These reactive oxygen species do have a purposeful role in spermatozoan capacitation, the acrosomal reaction and binding to gametocyte. Nonparticulate radiation emitted from the mobile phones ends up in reactive oxygen species that cause DNA polymer fragmentation; so decreasing motility and viability of spermatozoan. There is vital association between oligozoospermia abnormalities with the occupation hazards. Azoospermia is seen in Klinefelter's syndrome, hypogonadotrophic hypogonadism, ductal obstruction or in case of agenesis of vas deferens. Oligospermia is seen in anatomic defects of male procreative tract, in endocrinopathies and with genetic disorders. Abnormal seminal volume is seen in retrograde ejaculation, infection, ejaculatory failure. Abnormal morphology of spermatozoon is seen in varicocoele, stress and infection. Immunological factors, infection, defect in spermatozoan structure, varicocoele is related to abnormal motility of spermatozoan.[11]

The genetic landscape of male sterility is highly complex as male reproductive gland histologic phenotypes are extremely heterogeneous and multiple genes are concerned with gametogenesis. Approximately 50% cases of male infertility are idiopathic. Most of the idiopathic cases are found to be genetic origin as a result of multiple genes concerned with gametogenesis.[12] The genes concerned are cystic fibrosis transmembrane conductance regulator gene mutations of which cystic fibrosis, absence of vas deferens and sex hormone receptor gene whose mutations cause the sex hormone unfitness syndrome and spermatogenic damage. Chromosomal anomalies and microdeletions of the azoospermia factor region of the Y chromosome are common causes. Sex chromosome aneuploidies such as 47XXY, 47XYY are the foremost common chromosomal anomalies in infertile men. Y chromosome microdeletions are etiological factors for idiopathic azoospermia. Genetic factors are contributive to male sterility is in azoospermia, however, the numbers of known genetic anomalies are perpetually growing. Lifestyle factors such as smoking cigarettes, alcohol intake, use of illicit medication, obesity, psychological stress, advanced paternal age, dietary practices, lack of sleep and radiation exposure are contributive factors for sterility. Obesity concurrently contributes to hypogonadism and male subfertility. Obesity is related to leptin resistance, it is possible that leptin deficiency contribute to obesity-induced hypogonadism.[12]

Environmental exposure to industrial wastes, chemicals, harmful substances would lead to poor ejaculate quality, injury to sperm cell deoxyribonucleic acid (DNA) integrity. DNA fragmentation is also used as a marker for exposure to toxicants and a diagnostic tool for male infertility. Air pollution being world's largest environmental health risk. There has been a robust association of pollution levels with abnormal sperm cell shape.[13]

Adult testicular issues, as well as poor ejaculate quality and sex gland cell cancer are thought to be late onset symptoms of biological failure of the genital system. These biological process failures might be the result of genetic and environmental factors. There are many levels of sperm cell chromatin granule abnormalities like loss of physical integrity, loss of deoxyribonucleic acid strand breaks, altered tertiary chromatin granule configuration which are seen with environmental stress, sequence mutations and chromosomal abnormalities which could ultimately cause abnormal chromatin granule structure incompatible with fertility. Another mechanism of sperm cell deoxyribonudeic acid injury is unsuccessful caspase-mediated cell death by the expression of Fas substance. Syndromes related to severely impaired ejaculate quality resembling XXY-syndrome and different disorders of sexual development have a well-defined genetic origin. Male infertility attributable to poor ejaculate quality could be a symptom of disorder of sexual development, however, it is neither an isolated pathological entity nor a diagnosis. Semen profile with low sperm cell count, high frequency of abnormal sperm cell and poor sperm cell motility may well be related to chromosomal translocations and undiagnosed seminoma.[14]

Future analysis within the space of subfertility/infertility also will assist in finding innovations for brand new strategies of birth control and in facilitating to resolve problems with recurrent spontaneous miscarriages. Due to rise in lifestyle-related infertility such as excessive smoking, stress, radiations and exposure to pollution, the demand and use of fertility services can increase at a big pace. The scientific advancement of motor-assisted reproductive technologies will also contribute to augmented adoption of those services.

REFERENCES

1. www.who.int. Sterility may be a world public health issue. 2018.

2. Martin JA, Hamilton BE, Sutton PD, Ventura SJ, Menacker F, Kirmeyer S. Births; Final knowledge for 2004. Natl important Stat Rep 2006; 55:1–101.

3. Sadock BJ, Sadock VA. 9th ed. Philadelphia: Lippincott Williams and Wilkins; Kaplans and Sadocks Symptoms of medicine behavioural Sciences Clinical Psychiatry 2003;872–4.

4. Mascarenhas MN1, Flaxman SR, Boerma T, Vanderpoel S, Stevens GA. National, regional, and world trends in sterility prevalence since 1990: a scientific analysis of 277 health surveys. PLoS Med 2012;9(12):e1001356.

5. Kumar D. Prevalence of feminine sterility and its socio-economic factors in social group communities of central Bharat. Rural Remote Health 2007;7(2);456.

6. Adamson PC, Krupp K, Freeman AH, Klausner JD, Arthur L. Prevalence and correlates of primary sterility among young girls in Mysore, India. Indian J MEd Res 2011;134(4):440.

7. Kumar TCA. Fertility and in-vitro fertilization in Bharat. Curr Sci 2004;86:254–6.

8. Plachot M, Belaisch-Allart J, Mayenga JM, Chouraqui A, Tesquier L, Serkine AM. Outcome of standard IVF and ICSI on relation oocytes in delicate male issue sterility. Hum Reprod 2002; 17:362–9.

9. Harris ID, Fronczak C, Roth L, Meacham RB. Fertility and therefore the aging male. Rev Urol 2011;13:e184–90.

10. Miyamoto T, Tsujimura A, Miyagawa Y, Koh E, Namiki M, Sengoku K. Male sterility and its causes in Human. Adv Urol 2012;2012:384520.

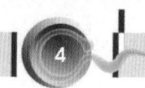

11. Al-Quzwini OF, Al-Taee HA, Al-Shaikh SF. Male sterility and its association with activity and portable towers hazards: Associate in Nursing analytic study. Mideast Fertility Society Journal 2016,21(4):237–9.

12. Plaseska-Karanfilska, Noveski P, Moneva Z. Genetic causes of Male sterility. Balkan J MEd Genet 2012;15:31–4.

13. Schulte RT, Ohl DA, Smith GD. Spermatozoan polymer injury in male infertility: etiologies, assays and outcomes. J Assit Reprod Genet 2010;27(1):3–12.

14. Juul A, Almstrup K, Andersson AM, Jensen TK, Jorgensen N, Main KM, et. al. Doable foetal determinants of male sterility. Nat Rev Endocrinol 2014 Sep;10(9):553–62.

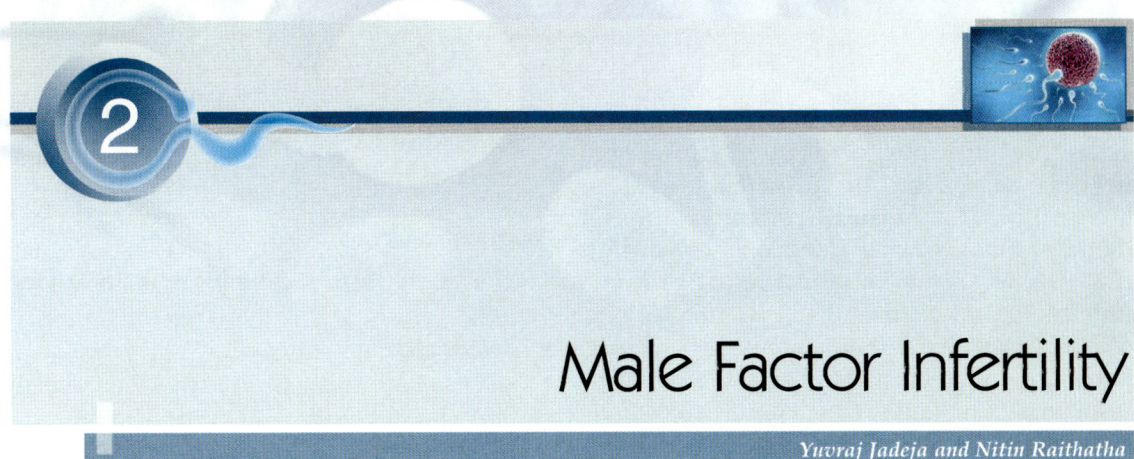

Male Factor Infertility

Yuvraj Jadeja and Nitin Raithatha

The definition of infertility as per World Health Organization (WHO) includes the inability of sexually active couple (at least three times per month) not using contraception to achieve pregnancy within a year. The prevalence of infertility is on a constant rise, male infertility shares a major burden of that load. Although an abnormal semen analysis is the only glaring indicator of underlying male infertility, other factors may also play a role, even when semen analysis is normal.[1]

Development of Male Reproductive Axis

The hypothalamus is the most crucial processing epicentre and plays a vital role in complex coordination of homeostatic mechanisms and functions related to development and reproduction. The hypothalamic-pituitary-gonadal axis (HPO) plays pivotal role in fertility among males via a complex feed forward/back entity mechanism. The gonadotropin-releasing hormone (GnRH) is secreted by hypothalamus and acts on the pituitary gland to produce Luteinizing Hormone (LH) and Follicle Stimulating Hormone (FSH). Within the testis testosterone production is regulated by effects of LH on Leydig cells, while FSH induces spermatogenesis in Sertoli cells. The release of GnRH and pituitary secretion of LH and FSH are in turn, controlled by levels of sex hormones, i.e. testosterone and estrogen and FSH stimulated inhibin[2] (Fig. 2.1).

Spermatogenesis

Spermatogenesis compromise of four key steps that occur in the seminiferous epithelium. These steps include spermatogonial proliferation and differentiation, meiosis of spermatogonial proliferation and differentiation, meiosis of spermatocytes, spermiogenesis and spermiation. On an average, the duration of spermatogenesis in humans is 74 days.[3]

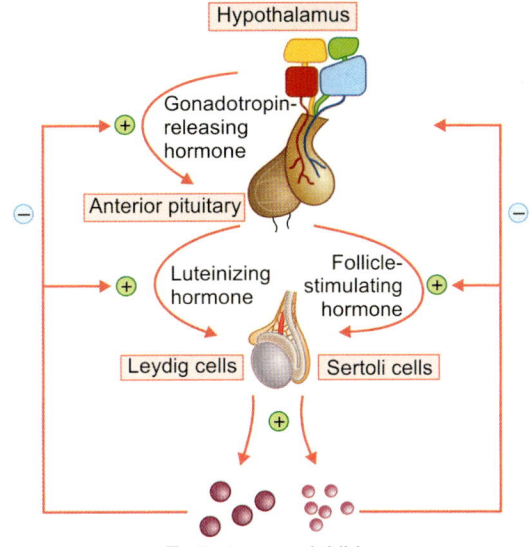

Fig. 2.1: Male hypothalamic-pituitary-gonadal axis.

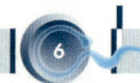

Risk Factors and Consequences

There are multiple factors that can cause reduced male fertility, and these include congenital or acquired urogenital abnormalities, malignancies, infections, endocrine disturbances, genetic abnormalities, and immunological factors.[4] The common causes of male infertility from the analysis of 10,469 patients have been listed in Table 2.1.[5] Finding from an Indian study, which analysed semen samples from 240 male partners of couple seeking consultation for infertility indicated that abnormal semen parameters were significantly higher among those exposed to lifestyle and/or environmental factors compared to those not exposed. The study findings further indicated that the risk of declining semen quality, decreased antioxidants levels, and greater sperm DNA damage were greater among those exposed to various lifestyles factors, such as tobacco

smoking, chewing and alcohol use, as well as exposure to toxic agents, compared to those unexposed to these factors.[6]

Prognostic Factors

The key prognostic factors for male infertility include:[4]
- Duration of infertility.
- Causes of infertility (primary or secondary).
- Age and fertility status of the female partner.
- Abnormalities in semen parameters.

Types of Male infertility

Male infertility can be classified into three major types (Table 2.2)[8]
1. **Non-obstructive infertility:** Caused due to inadequate sperm production by testes, observed in 60% of cases.
2. **Obstructive infertility:** Caused due to the presence of blockage in the genital tract, observed in 38% of cases.
3. **Coital infertility:** Caused due to sexual dysfunction, caused by impaired intromission or ejaculation observed in 2% of cases.

Unexplained Male Infertility: Uncommon Condition

Male infertility can be further classified into idiopathic male infertility (IMI) and unexplained male infertility (UMI). A threefold higher prevalence of IMI is generally observed when compared to UMI. The differentiating features between these two types is a normal physical examination and endocrine testing

Table 2.1: Causes of male infertility—associated factors	
Male infertility—associated factors	Percentage
Idiopathic	31
Maldescended	7.8
Infection	8
Disorders of semen deposition and sexual factors	5.9
Systemic disease	3.1
Varicocele	15.6
Endocrine	8.9
Immunologic	4.5
Obstructions	1.7
Other	5.5

Table 2.2: Causes of different types of male infertility		
Causes of non-obstructive infertility	Causes of obstructive infertility	Causes of coital infertility
• Hormonal abnormalities	• Congenital absence of vas defrences	• Erectile dysfunction
• Genetic causes	• Vasectomy	• Premature ejaculation
• Varicocele	• Vasal obstruction	• Penile deformities
• Exposure to gonadotoxins	• Epididymal obstruction	• Anejaculation
• Orchitis	• Ejaculatory duct obstruction	• Retrograde ejaculation
• Testicular torsion, trauma, tumours		
• Autoimmune infertility		

with abnormal semen parameters in IMI compared to UMI, where an evaluation will yield a normal semen analysis and physical exam in the absence of female factor.[9]

Etiologies of Unexplained Male Infertility

Immune Infertility: Antisperm antibodies (ASA) production is a key factor involved in the development of immune infertility caused due to a breach in blood testis barrier by previous trauma, infection and/or obstruction. Hamada et al reported that these antibodies are common occurrence in men with unexplained infertility (42%), men undergoing fertility evaluations (10.7%), and in men of couples undergoing *in vitro* fertilization (10%) in comparison to fertile men (2%). Immunoglobulin class A and G and their presence confers decreased fertilization capability.

A recent systemic review/meta analysis by Ciu et al. which assessed the association of ASA and basic semen parameters in infertile men, indicated that ASA positive patients had lower sperm concentrations, longer semen liquefaction time and reduced sperm motility when compared to ASA negative controls. Studies also indicate ASA may be associated with sperm agglutination and clumping. However, normal semen parameters may also be present with immune related infertility.[9]

Reactive Oxygen Species

Reactive oxygen species (ROS) are produced in human semen predominantly by leukocytes and immature spermatozoa. There are two primary pathways which are implicated in generation of ROS. The first is at the level of sperm plasma membrane via the NADPH oxidase systems, and the second is at the mitochondrial level by the NADH dependent oxidoreductase system. Raised ROS causes decreased motility and failure of sperm oocyte fusion by damaging proteins, DNA, and biomembranes in sperm structures.[10,11] Estimates indicate that nearly 40–80% of infertile men have elevated oxidative stress. Factors that aggravate the accumulation of inflammatory cells in the genital tract include infections or smoking and conditions such as

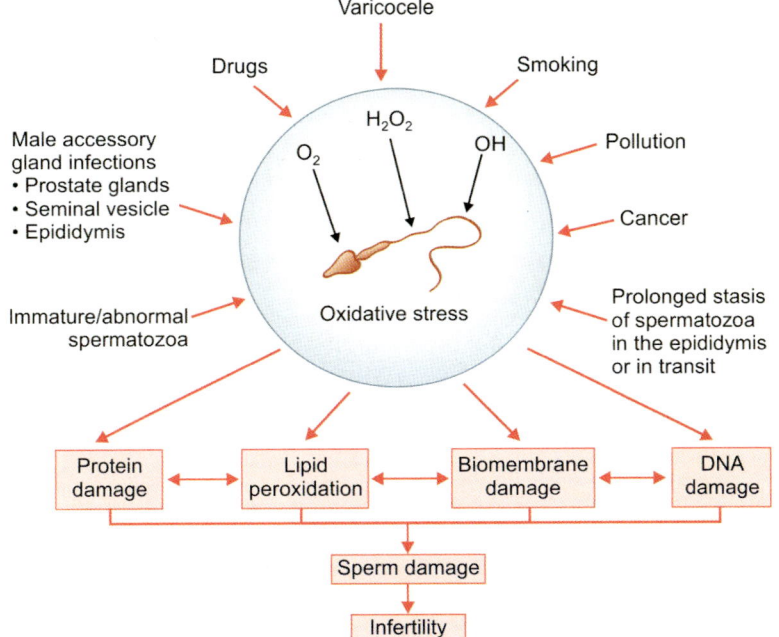

Fig. 2.2: Outcomes of oxidative stress in relation to male infertility.

varicocele which lead to production of imma-ture cells (Fig. 2.2).

In leukocytes, ROS is generated under conditions of infection and inflammation and activated leukocytes are capable of producing 100 times higher amounts of ROS than inactivated leukocytes. Recent evidence indicates presence of low levels of leukocyto spermia (below 1 million WBC/1 milliliter of semen) as harmful and correcting it may result in improved pregnancy rates.

Genetic Defects

Infertility in men can occur as a result of genetic damage, including the alternation of spermatogenesis and/or sperm function. In a study of 2650 (5300 patients) who underwent chromosome analysis before ICSI, male patients were found to harbour more frequent chromosomal abnormalities compared to females which includes abnormal karyotypes with abnormal sex chromosomes and auto-somal aberrations.[12] Cystic fibrosis gene mutations and Y microdeletion are other two common genetic factor involved (Table 2.3).

Components of Complete Evaluation for Male Infertility

Multiple factors can lead to male infertility, however, not all of these can be identified and managed effectively. Therefore, it is of paramount importance to recognise and treat correctable conditions (Table 2.4).[13]

Physical Examination

A physical examination should include examination of penis, location of urethral meatus, palpation and measurement of testes, presence and consistency of both vasa and epididymis, the presence/absence of a varico-cele, secondary sex characteristics. The Praders orchidometer is used for measuring the testicular volume commonly, the diagnosis of varicocele is generally done based on a physical examination.

Semen Analysis

Semen analysis is crucial for diagnosis and assessment of severity of male infertility. A standardized set of instructions should be provided by physicians, including details of defined pretest abstinence interval of 2–5 days prior to semen collection. Basic parameters analyzed in a standard semen analysis including pH, volume, concentration, morphology and motility. The WHO Laboratory Manual for Examination and Processing of Human Semen has provided lower limits of the accepted reference values for semen analysis (Table 2.5).[13]

Other Procedure and Tests for Assessing Male Infertility

Indications for hormonal evaluation include:[14]
1. Men with abnormal semen parameters, especially when sperm concentration is <10 million/ml.

Table 2.3: Recommended tests for genetic screening and their indications[7]	
Indications	Recommended tests
Men with infertility of unknown etiology and sperm concentration <5 million/ml who are candidates for ART	Y microdeletion and G band karyotyping
Nonobstructive azoospermia in a male considering testicular sperm retrieval for ART.	Y microdeletion and G band karyotyping
Azoospermic or oligozoospermic men with the absence of at least one vas deferens at physical examination.	CFTR gene mutation analysis
History of recurrent miscarriage or personal/familiar history of genetic syndromes.	G band karyotyping

Table 2.4: Major aspect of history taking in male infertility

1. Infertility history

- Age of partner, time attempting to conceive.
- Contraceptive method and duration.
- Previous pregnancies (same partner/other partner).
- Previous treatment.
- Treatment evaluation of female partner.

2. Sexual history

- Potency, libido, lubricant use
- Ejaculation, timed intercourse

3. Childhood and development cryptorchidism, hernia, testicular trauma/torsion/infection (mumps)

- Sexual development, puberty onset

4. Personal history

- Systemic diseases (diabetes, cirrhosis, hypertension), sexually transmitted diseases, tuberculosis, viral infections

5. Previous surgeries

- Orchidopexy, herniorrhaphy, orchiectomy (testicular cancer, torsion).
- Retroperitoneal and pelvic surgery.
- Other inguinal, scrotal and perineal surgery.
- Bariatric surgery, bladder neck surgery, transurethral resection of prostrate.

6. Gonadotoxin exposure

- Pesticides, alcohol, cocaine, marijuana abuse-medication (chemotherapy agents, cimetidine, sulfasalazine, finestaride, calcium blockers, alpha blockers).
- Organic solvents, heavy metals.
- Anabolic steroids, tobacco use.
- High temperature, electromagnetic energy.
- Radiation.

7. Family history

- Cystic Fibrosis, endocrine disease and infertility in the family

8. Current health status

- Respiratory infection
- Anosmia
- Galactorrhea
- Visual disturbances
- Obesity

Table 2.5: World Health Organization criteria for a normal semen analysis

Lower limits of the accepted reference values for semen analysis

Parameter	Reference values
On at least two occasions	
Ejaculate volume	1.5 ml
pH	7.2
Sperm concentration	15×10^6 spermatozoa/ml
Total sperm number	39×10^6 spermatozoa/ml
Percentage motility	40%
Forward progression	32%
Normal morphology	4%
Sperm agglutination	Absent
Viscosity	<2 cm thread after liquefication

Note: Data from WHO 2010[10] Practice Committee. Evaluation of the infertility male. Fertil Steri 2015.

2. Men with impaired sexual function
3. Men with other clinical findings that suggest a specific endocrinopathy.

There is no consensus on whether all infertile men should undergo a routine endocrine evaluation. Measurement of serum FSH and total testosterone (T) concentrations should be considered where indicated, and a more extensive evaluation should be considered if total T level is low (<300 ng/dL), which includes total testosterone levels, LH levels, FSH levels and prolactin with TSH (Table 2.6).

ULTRASOUND

Transrectal Ultrasound

Seminal vesicles are normally less than 1.5 cm in AP diameter. Transrectal ultrasonography can identify the presence of dilated seminal vesicles/ejaculatory ducts and/or midline prostrate cystic structures, which are indicative of complete or partial ejaculatory duct obstruction. In patients with complete ejaculatory duct obstruction, low volume, fructose negative, acidic and azoospermic features are often observed. Patients with CBAVD have

Table 2.6: Relationship between testosterone, LH, FSH and Prolactin with clinical correlation

Basal Hormone levels in various clinical states

Clinical conditions	FSH	LH	T	PRL
Normal spermatogenesis	Normal	Normal	Normal	Normal
Hypo hypo	Low	Low	Low	Normal
Abnormal spermatogenesis	High/normal	Normal	Normal	Normal
Hyper Hypo/Complete testicular failure	High	High	Normal/low	Normal
PRL secreting tumor	Normal/low	Normal/low	Low	High

absent or atrophic seminal vesicles as observed using TRUS. Low volume semen, oligoasthenospermia, and poor forward progression may be observed in men partial ejaculatory duct obstruction.[14]

Scrotal Ultrasound

A physical examination provides a clue to origin of most scrotal pathologies, such as varicoceles, spermatoceles, absence of the vasa, epididymal induration, and testicular masses. However, scrotal ultrasonography may be helpful in cases where physical examination is indeterminate. Furthermore, vague findings on physical examination may be clarified by scrotal ultrasonography, such as small scrotal ultrasonography, such as small scrotal sacs, testes being present in the upper scrotum, and other findings that preclude a physical examination of the scrotum.[14]

Specialized Clinical Tests on Semen and Sperm

Specialized clinical tests may be useful in cases where semen analyses have failed to accurately diagnose infertility. Such tests are generally considered for men in whom the identification of the cause of infertility will likely help in directing adequate treatment.
- Strict sperm morphology.
- Sperm fragmentation and DNA integrity.
- Quantitation of leukocytes in semen.
- Antisperm antibodies.
- Oxidative stress.
- Sperm viability.
- Sperm aneuploidy testing.

A detailed work-up plan for unexplained, male infertility and management scenarios has been described in Fig. 2.3.

ASSISTED REPRODUCTION FOR MALE INFERTILITY

Assisted reproductive techniques (ART) are becoming increasingly popular as adjective treatments for managing male factor infertility. In a couple in whom the female partner has a normal fertility status and at least 3×10^6 progressively motile spermatozoa are recovered after sperm preparation, IUI may be considered first-line treatment.

In Vitro Fertilization

Optimized IVF may be proposed to couples if pregnancy is not achieved after 3–6 cycles of IUI.

Intracytoplasmic Sperm Injection

Indications for performing ICSI includes flagellar dyskinesia, immotile cilia syndromes, globozoospermia, and presence of significant levels of antisperm antibodies. Intracytoplasmic sperm injection should be considered when there are $<0.5 \times 10^6$ of progressively motile spermatozoa after seminal fluid processing or in sperm recovered surgically from the testis or epididymis.

OTHER MODALITIES

Donor Insemination

This can be considered as an alternative when all the above treatment options have failed.

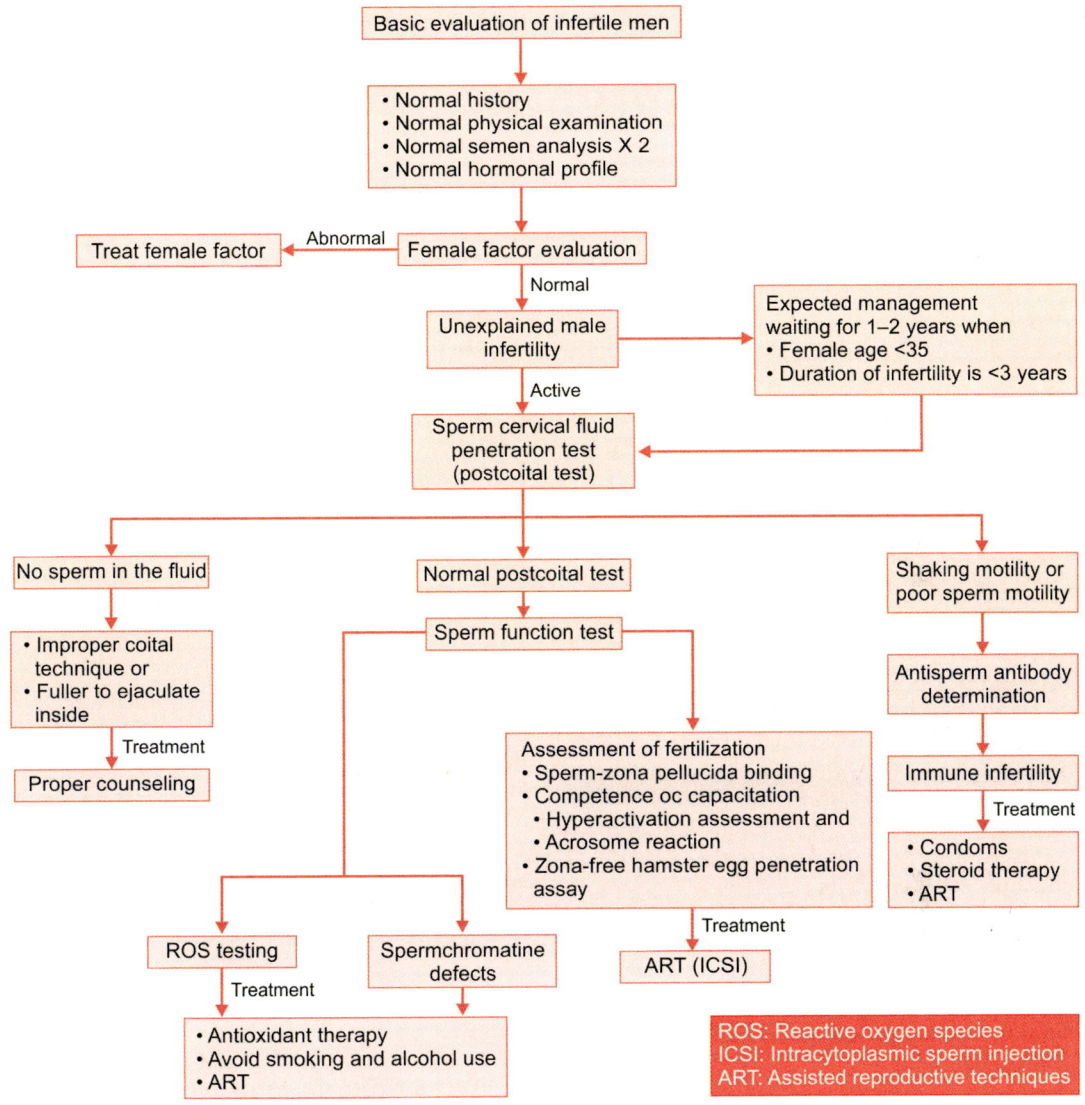

Fig. 2.3: Work up plan for male infertility.

Surgical Treatment Options

Varicocele Repair

Though the benefits of this repair in fertility remains controversial, though there are reports of improved semen parameters following treatment. No benefits in men with normal semen parameters and subclinical varicosele.

Microsurgery/Vasovasostomy and Epididymovasostomy

Absolute indication for these reconstruction surgeries in Obstuctive Azoospermia.

PESA/MESA

In instances where reconstruction cannot be performed or is unsuccessful, PESA/MESA is recommended.

TESA/ Mapping/ Micro TESE

In patients with non obstructive azoospermia these modalities have been proved to be useful to retrieve sperms for ICSI even in the rarest of cases.

Transurethral incision of ejaculatory ducts or midline prostatic cysts could be used for distal obstruction in genital tracts in selected cases.

Counselling of Patients with Male Infertility

Anxiety, guilt and depression are common amongst men dealing with infertility. Every physician must play a vital role in counselling both partners and should update them with all available options. The partners should be counselled on lifestyle changes, alignment of intercourse with ovulation timings.

The treating physician should be mindful of giving false hopes to couples at the same time, should maintain a balance in providing them support and positivity.

REFERENCES

1. American Urological Association. The optimal evaluation of the infertile male. AUA Best practice Statement 2010.
2. Whirledge S, Cidlowski JA. Glucocorticoids, stress, and fertility. Minerva Endocrinol 2010; 35(2):109–25.
3. Amann R. The cycle of the seminiferous epithelium in human: A need to revisit? J Andrology. 2008;29:469–87.
4. Jungwirth A, Diemer T, Dohle GR. European Association of Urology. Male Infertiltiy 2013.
5. Jungwirth A, Giwercman A, Tournaye H. European Association of Urology Guidelines on Male Infertiltiy: The 2012 Update Eur Urol 2012; 62(2):324–32.
6. Kumar S, Muraka S, MishraVV. Environmental and lifestyles factors in deterioration of male reproductive health. Indian J Med Res 2014; 140(Suppl1):S29–S35.
7. Esteves SC. An update on the clinical assessment of the infertile male. Clinics 2011;66(4):691–700.
8. Raheem AA. Male infertility: Causes and investigations. Trends in Urology Mens Health 2011.
9. Hamada A. Unexplained Male infertility: Diagnosis and Management. Int Baz J Urol 2012;38: 576–95.
10. Agarwal A, Sekhon LH. The role of antioxidants therapy in the treatment of male infertility. Human Fertility 2010;13(4):217–25.
11. Cocuzza M, Sikka SC, Athayde KS. Clinical relevance of oxidative stress and sperm chromatin damage in male infertility: An evidence based analysis. Int Braz J Urol 2007; 33(5): 603–21.
12. Kayed HF, Mansour RT, Aboulghar MA. Screening for chromosomal abnormalities in 2650 infertile couples undergoing ICSI. Reprod Biomed Online 2006;12(3):359–70.
13. ASRM. Diagnostic evaluation of the infertile male: a committee opinion. Fertil Steril 2012; 98:294–301.
14. Esteves SC, Hamada A, Kondaray V, et al. What every gynaecologists should know about male infertility. Arch Gynaecol Obstet. 2012;286: 217–29.

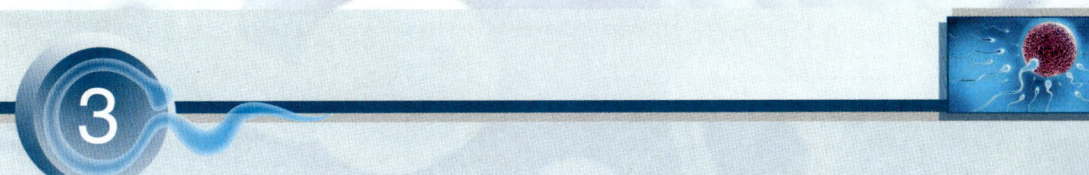

Exercise, Lifesytle and Nutrition Role in Male Infertility

Atul Munshi

Introduction

Infertility is defined as the inability of a couple to conceive after 1 year of attempting pregnancy. According to the CDC, in the United States, 10.9% of women aged 15–44 have impaired fertility. Men are responsible for this problem at least 40–50% percent of the time. There are many factors that can affect **male fertility**, among which **lifestyle choices** play a key role. **Nutrition and physical activity and exercise are also important.**

Incidence

Among infertile couples, it is man who is responsible for 50% cases of infertility. The studies indicate that 6% of men aged 15–44 years are infertile or their fertility is significantly compromised.[1] Reports in recent years have shown that incidence of male infertility has increased as a result of various factors such as environmental pollution, stress and lifestyle.[2]

Prevalence of primary infertility in India, according to WHO, is estimated to be between 3.9 and 16.8%. Overall, up to 12% of men of reproductive age suffer from male infertility.

Discussion

Living a healthy **lifestyle** is important to our fertility. Lifestyle factors can affect a man's fertility, and many of these factors are things that a man can control. Leading a healthy lifestyle improves not only your chances of conceiving but also your overall health.

Psychological Stress

Many forms of stress including psychological can affect male fertility and reproduction. The autonomic nervous system and the adrenal hormones participate in the classic stress response while also affecting the reproductive system. Evidence exists that mild-to-severe emotional stress decreases testosterone and interferes with spermatogenesis in the human male.[3] It has been observed that some seminal antioxidant contents, as well as motility and morphologically normal spermatozoa decrease in students undergoing examination stress.[4] Further, reports indicate that work stress disturbs the LH pulse, which is responsible for erectile dysfunction and poor semen quality.[5]

Genital Heat Stress

Normal sperm production depends on an optimal testicular temperature maintained below body temperature (typically between 34 and 35°C).[2] The temperature range for spermatogenesis is critical such that lower temperature reduces metabolic rate and sperm can be stored for longer.[6] It is well known that the increased temperature of the scrotum affects spermatogenesis.

Too tight clothing, long sitting in heated environment and too much use of computer and laptops may have adverse effect.

Smoking

Cigarettes contain more than 4000 chemical compounds and at least 400 toxic substances. The effect of smoking on infertility and sexual dysfunction is rarely described. As a result, awareness about these additional ill effects of smoking is limited. The harmful effects of cigarette smoking on human male fertility are now clear. The association of smoking and male sexual dysfunction has been found in both epidemiologic and clinical studies. Available evidence suggests an association between smoking and erectile dysfunction.[7]

PASSIVE SMOKING IS EQUALLY HARMFUL

Alcoholism

Excessive Alcohol intake has long been associated with reproductive health disorders such as impotence or testicular atrophy. In men, alcohol reduces testosterone levels. A report showed that testosterone levels fell just after five days among normal healthy men who were given alcohol and continued to fall throughout the four-week study period.[8] Excessive alcohol consumption has therefore been linked to the production of abnormal sperm cells with deformed heads and tails.[8]

Occupational Causes

Data on occupational hazards to male reproduction remain controversial. Exposure to heavy metals such as cadmium, lead, arsenic and zinc has been reported to impair spermatogenesis, although the data are conflicting.[9,10] Certain pesticides and herbicides have more clearly been shown to be toxic to spermatogenesis,[11] as have some organic chemicals.[12] The role of occupational exposure to heat is well documented.

Environmental Causes

Data on environmental factors and infertility in the male are also controversial. There would seem to be clear evidence that occupational or environmental exposure to heat will have adverse consequences for spermatogenesis[13], and will prolong time to pregnancy.[14]

Role of Nutrition in Male Infertility

There is a definitive role of nutrition in causative factor for male infertility. Long-term dietary factor deficiency can lead to irreversible damage.

During the last decade there has been a huge improvement in the explanation of spermatozoa pathophysiological processes and therefore in the nutraceutical treatments. Unfortunately, there are no clinical trials that demonstrate as secondary and tertiary outcomes pregnancy rate and miscarriage rate respectively.

A dietary pattern that includes fruits and vegetables is rich in **antioxidants** such as vitamin E, vitamin C, and beta carotene. Numerous health benefits have been ascribed to antioxidants, mainly because they protect against generation of reactive oxygen species. The production of reactive oxygen species has the potential to negatively affect sperm motility and the capacity for sperm–oocyte fusion. Moreover, antioxidants are thought to have the ability to protect human spermatozoa against endogenous oxidative damage by neutralizing hydroxyl, superoxide, and hydrogen peroxide radicals and preventing sperm agglutination.

A positive association of **fish intake** with sperm concentration and morphology could be mediated through increased intake of long-chain n-3 fatty acids. Sperm and testes have a higher concentration of long-chain polyunsaturated fatty acids (PUFAs), especially docosahexaenoic acid (DHA), compared with other cells or tissues in the human body. The structural integrity of the spermatozoa cell membrane plays a pivotal role in successful fertilization.

Deleterious effects of many dietary factors can impair spermatogenesis, reduce sperm concentration and motility, and increase sperm DNA damage, especially in infertile obese men with diabetes, dyslipidemia, or metabolic syndrome.

Role of Calcium and Vitamin D in Male Infertility

- Vitamin D deficiency and low ionized calcium are linked with semen quality and sex steroid levels in infertile men.
- Vitamin D receptors and vitamin D metabolic enzymes are expressed in male reproductive system, suggesting that vitamin D_3 plays a pivotal role in male reproductive biology.
- Results of animal models and cross-sectional cohort studies have suggested a beneficial role for vitamin D in male reproduction.
- Vitamin D is important for spermatogenesis and maturation of human spermatozoa.
- Infertile men with vitamin D deficiency had lower sperm motility, total numbers of motile sperm, inhibin B, sex-hormone-binding-globulin and testosterone/estradiol ratio.
- Associations between vitamin D deficiency and low calcium with semen quality and sex steroids support the existence of a cross-link between regulators of calcium homeostasis and gonadal function in infertile men.
- **Vitamin D was shown to be positively associated to sperm motility**, and to exert direct actions on spermatozoa, including modulation of intracellular calcium homeostasis and activation of molecular pathways involved in sperm motility, capacitation and acrosome reaction.
- **There is positive impact of vitamin D supplementation on live birth rate** and serum inhibin B in oligozoospermic and vitamin D-deficient men may be of clinical importance and warrant verification by others.

Undernutrition poses adverse effect on the reproductive capacity of males. The restriction of nutrient intake or deficiency of particular nutrients in experimental animals delays sexual maturity and causes rapid regressive changes in male accessory organs. Therefore, successful reproduction requires complete provisions of macro- and micronutrients, including zinc, vit A (retinol), vit B_{12}, vit B_9, vit E, vit D, folate, selenium, nickel, manganese, chromium, copper, fatty acid, protein, arginine, and carnitine.[15]

Exercise

Role of exercise in male infertility is again a controversial topic. Moderate exercise may be beneficial for patients. However, prolonged, excessive exercise may be just as bad as no exercise at all. So, the key is, as with most things, moderation. Adequate daily rest is equally important.

Other Studies for Exercise

Overall, none of the semen parameters were materially associated with regular exercise. Compared with no regular exercise, bicycling 5 hrs/week was associated with low sperm concentration. These associations did not vary appreciably by age, body mass index, or history of male factor infertility.

Although the study suggests no overall association between regular physical activity and semen quality, bicycling 5 hrs/week was associated with lower sperm concentration and TMS.[16]

Current Recommendation

Counselling Plays an Important Role

'Lifestyle' factors can impair semen quality, e.g. heavy smoking, alcohol abuse, use of anabolic steroids, extreme sports (marathon training, excessive strength sports), and an increase in scrotal temperature through thermal underwear, sauna or hot tub use, or occupational exposure to heat sources. A considerable number of drugs can affect spermatogenesis.

Encourage a healthy lifestyle: There are several things a man can do to optimize his sperm production and quality. Sperm production takes 75 to 90 days. Avoiding harmful substances, medications, or lifestyles should occur in advance of attempting pregnancy. You should review your medical history and all current medications and supplements you take with your physician. Stress may contribute to altered sperm production.

Avoid smoking: Several studies have clearly shown that cigarette smoking lowers both sperms count and sperm motility. If you or your partner smokes, now is the time to quit!

Avoid alcohol and drug use: Excessive alcohol consumption has clearly been shown to impair normal sperm. The evidence regarding moderate alcohol intake is less clear, but most experts agree it is best for patients to avoid more than 1 drink per day. There is some evidence that even moderate drinking (1 drink every other day) may decrease IVF success. Other drugs such as marijuana have been shown to affect sperm parameters and should be avoided.

Avoid excessive heat: It is well known that the testicles should be cooler than the rest of the body for sperm production to be at its best. The harmful effect of a varicocele on sperm production is believed to result from the extra warming of the area caused by the dilated veins. There is no scientific evidence to support the claim that boxer style shorts are better than briefs. It is advisable to avoid regular and prolonged exposure to the groin area with sources of heat exposure such as hot tubs, saunas, and laptop computers.

Identify and avoid environmental hazards: If patient's work or hobby brings him into contact with environmental dangers such as heavy metals like cadmium or lead, pesticides, solvents, organic fumes, or radiation exposure, he may be unknowingly affecting his fertility by impairing sperm production.

Limit caffeine: Limit coffee or other caffeine containing beverages to 1 or 2 drinks per day.

Proper diet/weight: Eating a balanced diet is important. Extra fruits and vegetables along with plenty of fluids is a good idea. It is probably best to avoid high intake of soy products, since they can contain weak plant estrogens. Men who are overweight should begin a weight loss program.

Exercise: Moderate exercise may be beneficial for patients. However, prolonged, excessive exercise may be just as bad as no exercise at all. So, the key is, as with most things, moderation. Adequate daily rest is equally important.

Overall male infertility is reasonable manageable provided lifestyle management, nutrition and regular exercise is taken care of.

REFERENCES

1. Smith JF, Walsh TJ. Sexual, marital and social impact of a man's perceived infertility diagnosis. J Sex Med 2009;6(9):2505–15.
2. Mendiola J, Torres-contero AM, et al. Lifestyle factors and male infertility: an evidence-based review. Arch Med Sci 2009;5(1A):S3–S12.
3. Hall E, Burt VK. Male fertility: psychiatric considerations. 2012,97(2):434–9.
4. Lampiao F Malawi. Variation of semen parameters in healthy medical students due to exam stress. Med J 2009;21(4):166–7.
5. Negro-Vilar. Stress and Other Environmental Factors Affecting Fertility in Men and Women: Overview. Environ Health Persp 1997;101(Suppl. 2):59–64.
6. Ivell R. Lifestyle impact and the biology of the human scrotum. Reprod Bio. Endocrinol 2009; 5:15.
7. Kumar N. The association between smoking and male fertility and sexual health. Indian J. Cancer 47:107–8.
8. Emanuele MA, et al. Alcohol and the Male Reproductive System. Alcohol Research & Health 2001;25(4):282–7.
9. Coste J Mandereaul, et al. Lead-exposed workmen and fertility: a cohort study. Eur J Epidemiol 1991,7:154–8.
10. Hu WY, Wu SH, et al. Toxicological ad epidemiological study on reproductive functions of male workers exposed to lead. J. Hygeine, Epidemiol Microbiol Immunol 1992,36:25–30.

11. Eaton M, Schenker M. Seven year follow up of workers exposed to 1,2 dibromo-3-chloropro-pane. J Occup Med 1986;28:1145–50.

12. Veulemans H, Steeno O, et al. Exposure to ethy-lene glycol ethers and spermatogemic disorders in man: a case control study. Br J Ind Med 1993; 50(1):71–80.

13. Mieusset R, Bujan L. Testicular Heating and its possible contributions to male infertility: a review. Int J Androl. 1995;18(4):169–84.

14. Thonneau P, Ducot B, et al. Heat exposure as a hazard to male fertility. Lancet 1996;347: 204–5.

15. Cheah Y, Yang W. Functions of essential nutri-tion for high quality spermatogenesis 2011;2: 182–97.

16. Wise LA, Craner DW, et. al. Physical activity and semen quality among men attending an inferti-lity clinic. Fertil Steril 2011;95(3):1025–30.

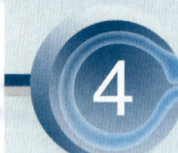
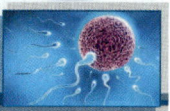

Imaging Modalities in Male Infertility

Amit Kharat, Nikith Somani and Jacob Jason

INTRODUCTION

Male infertility contributes to approximately 50% of infertile couples. The causes of male infertility can be pretesticular, testicular or post-testicular. A couple is termed infertile only after the couple engages in unprotected sexual intercourse for a period of 1 year without spontaneous induction of pregnancy. Hence, workup for infertility is done only after 12 months since the couple has attempted for conception.[1]

Evaluation of Male Infertility

The diagnostic workup should include the following:
1. Assessment of the medical history and physical evaluation
2. Assessment of semen and hormone analysis
3. Imaging modalities.

1. *Medical history and physical examination:* This should be mainly focused on identifying the risk factors that could affect fertility like age of the patient, sexual disorders, smoking history, frequency of sexual intercourse, etc.
2. *Semen and hormone analysis:* Normal semen should contain a volume >1.5 mm with concentration >15 million/ milliliter. Total progressive and non-progressive motility greater than 40%. If the ejaculate shows azoospermia, then laboratory analysis of FSH, LH can be used to distinguish between obstructive causes and non-obstructive causes.[2]

IMAGING

The main role of imaging is to identify causes such as congenital anomalies and diseases that obstruct the passage of sperms. The various imaging modalities that are routinely used include ultrasonography and magnetic resonance imaging.[3]

ULTRASONOGRAPHY

It is the most commonly preferred first line investigation since it is non-invasive, safe and inexpensive. Scrotal USG requires a high frequency linear array transducer (Fig. 4.1). Transrectal ultrasound is used to evaluate the

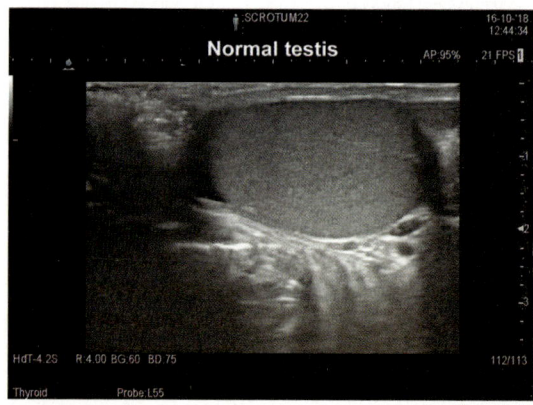

Fig. 4.1: This is a grey scale image of normal testes.

prostate and other causes of spermatic obstruction.[3]

MAGNETIC RESONANCE IMAGING

MRI is the most superior form of imaging. It is the modality of choice for accessory sex glands and their ducts.[3]

CAUSES OF MALE INFERTILITY

Pretesticular Causes

Imaging has limited role in evaluating pre testicular causes which are related to endo-crinopathies, chromosomal abnormalities or chronic medical conditions. They are more easily diagnosed with the help of biochemical and hormonal assessments or genetic testing. Some of the most common endocrinal disorders are described below.[4]

1. *Primary hypogonadism (hypergonado-tropic hypogonadism):* A typical example is Klinefelter's syndrome (Karyotype 47, XXY). They present with firm testes, tall stature, female hair distribution, obesity, diabetes mellitus, leukemia, germ cell tumors, infertility and gynecomastia. Testes show reduced volume, sclerosis and hyalinization of seminiferous tubules.[4]
2. *Secondary hypogonadism (Hypogonado-tropic hypogonadism):* A typical example is Kallman's syndrome which is due to mutation of KAL1 gene resulting in defi-ciency of GRH hormone secreted from hypothalamus. This indirectly leads to absent spermatogenesis and testosterone production.[5]
3. *Pituitary tumors:* The most common cause of infertility in pituitary tumors is that of prolactinoma resulting in hyperprolac-tinemia. The pulsatile secretion of GRH is inhibited by elevated prolactin levels resulting in spermatogenic arrest and impaired sperm motility and quality.[6]

TESTICULAR CAUSES

Varicocele: It is a common entity seen in the population, occurs due to abnormal dilation of pampiniform plexus. It is the most common treatable cause of male infertility. It is diagnosed mainly by clinical examination, with the patient standing and performing Valsalva maneuver. USG is used primarily for confirmation by checking the reflux of blood and dilated veins to at least 3 mm while doing Valsalva maneuver.[7] It can be graded as follows:

1. *Subclinical varicocele:* Neither palpable nor visible at rest or during Valsalva mane-uver, but visible on USG.[7]
   - Grade 1: Palpable during Valsalva mane-uver.
   - Grade 2: Palpable but not visible at rest.
   - Grade 3: Visible and palpable at rest.

   Left-sided varicoceles are more common since the left testicular vein drains directly into the left renal vein, as compared to the IVC, left renal vein has higher pressure. Hence, left renal vein is exposed to high pressure. An isolated right-sided varicocele should arise suspicion of retroperitoneal mass and undergo cross sectional imaging. The scrotum keeps the testes cooler as compared to the rest of the body. In vari-cocele, due to dilated veins, there is increased heat exchange resulting in higher temperatures in the scrotum. Hence, causing impaired spermatogenesis.[7]
2. *Intra-testicular varicocele:* It is similar to extra testicular varicocele and is diagnosed mainly by USG. There is dilatation of tubular intratesticular veins to a size larger than 2 mm. It usually lies close to the media-stinum. Color Doppler shows increased flow and reflux.[8]
3. *Testicular atrophy:* It is diagnosed when the volume of the testes is reduced by 50% of the normal side resulting in impaired spermatogenesis. Some of the causes include epididymo-orchitis, cryptorchi-dism, trauma, and varicocele.[9]
4. *Torsion* (Figs 4.2 and 4.5): It occurs due to the twisting of spermatic cord causing impaired venous flow and arterial ischemia. If not treated, leads to infarction

of testes. Bell-clapper deformity is a common risk factor for torsion. Here, there is abnormal insertion of tunica vaginalis allowing wide motility of the testes. It needs to be treated in 4–6 hours by detorsion to prevent ischemia. Detorsion should be done away from the midline and disappearance of pain is to be considered as a sign of successful detorsion. USG done after detorsion shows reduction in testes volume and decreased echogenicity and vascularity. However, the epididymis is not affected.[10]

5. *Orchitis and epididymo-orchitis* (Fig. 4.3): Inflammation of testes and epididymis can affect spermatogenesis and decrease the quality of sperm. It can also cause obstructive azoospermia which is secondary to infection/inflammation. USG shows increased testicular volume with heterogeneous echogenicity associated with enlarged heterogeneous epididymis.[11]

6. *Testicular microlithiasis* (Fig. 4.4): The seminiferous tubules show calcium deposits, USG-based diagnosis should depict 5 or more echogenic foci without posterior acoustic shadowing smaller than 3 mm per field of view. It is seen in cases of cryptorchidism, testicular atrophy, and hypogonadism. The cause of infertility in these cases is unclear.[12]

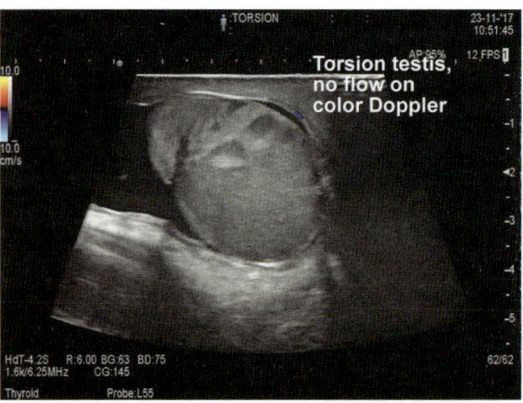

Fig. 4.2: This is a colour Doppler image of testes showing no flow with surrounding reactive hydrocele, features are suggestive of torsion testes.

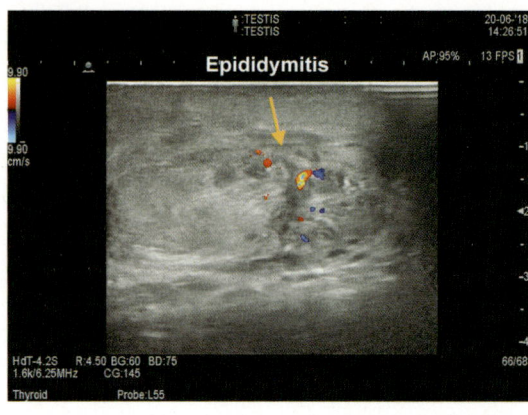

Fig. 4.3: This is a colour Doppler image showing bulky epididymis with increased vascularity, features suggestive of epididymitis.

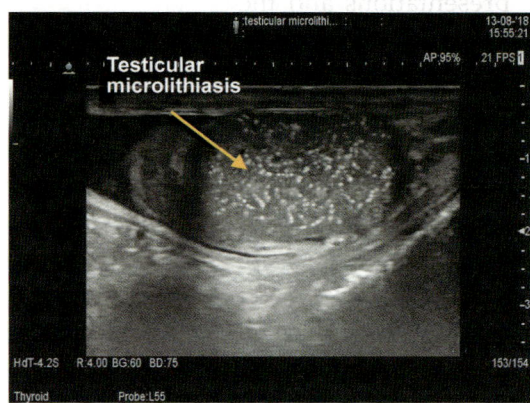

Fig. 4.4: This is a grey scale image of testes with multiple tiny echogenic calcifications within, features suggestive of microlithiasis.

7. *Cryptorchidism:* It is a common congenital abnormality of the male genitalia. It occurs due to delayed spontaneous descent of testes into the scrotal sac. After 6 months, spontaneous descent is highly unlikely. The fertility in these cases is inversely proportional to the age of the patient during surgery. The ectopic testes can be detected by scanning along the path of normal testicular decent. In cases of abdomino-pelvic testes, MRI is very useful modality for locating the testes. There is also a high incidence of testicular carcinoma in cases of cryptorchidism.[13]

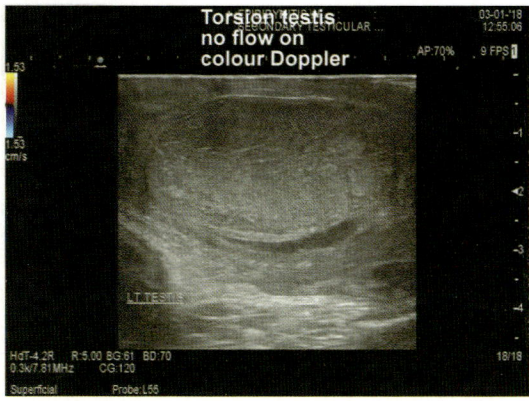

Fig. 4.5: This is a colour Doppler image of testes showing no flow, features are suggestive of torsion testes.

8. *Testicular cancer* (Fig. 4.6): It has variable presentations and the cause of infertility can include disruption of hypothalamic–pituitary–gonadal axis, immunological injury and systemic cancer related processes. Cancer treatment can also cause infertility due to the cytotoxic effects of radiation and chemotherapy. Most of testicular tumors show heterogenicity and hypoechogenicity compared to the surrounding testicular tissue with increased vascularity.[14]

POST-TESTICULAR CAUSES

It mainly includes congenital and acquired causes resulting in obstruction the ductal

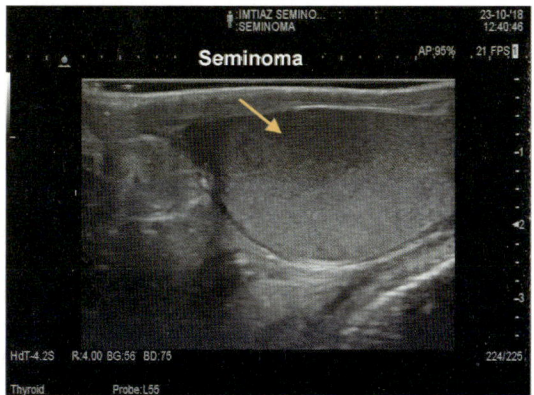

Fig. 4.6: A well-defined round to oval hypoechoic lesion with smooth margins noted within the testes, features suggestive of neoplastic origin.

system. Hence, the ducts which include ejaculatory ducts, seminal vesicle, epididymis, vas deferens and urethra should be evaluated carefully.[15]

Epididymal obstruction: These patients have azoospermia with normal ejaculate volume. Most common cause is epididymal infection, due to scarring and ultimately leading to obstruction.[15]

Vas deferens obstruction: Most common cause is vasectomy. It can also be related to surgeries such as hernia repair. USG typically shows dilated tubular ectasia.[15]

Ejaculatory duct obstruction: It is a rare cause of azoospermia and can be due to congenital condition (duct ectasia, stenosis, and prostatic cysts) and acquired conditions (infection, wrong catheterization, previous surgeries and stone formation at the level of ampulla). These patients have decreased ejaculatory force, hematospermia and pain during ejaculation.[16]

CYSTIC LESIONS

Ejaculatory duct cysts: These are thin walled paramedial cysts that develop in the Wolffian duct. Smaller ones are usually asymptomatic; however, larger cysts are symptomatic and can cause infertility due to obstruction.[17]

Cysts of Cowper gland ducts: Cowper glands secrete mucoid epithelium, providing alkalinity and lubrication for spermatozoa. When smaller, these are asymptomatic while larger cysts can cause various symptoms and infertility due to obstruction of bulbo-membranous portion of posterior urethra resulting in impaired ejaculation.[17]

Prostatic utricle and Müllerian duct cysts: These are midline prostatic cysts located behind the prostatic urethra. Prostatic utricle is often smaller as compared to Müllerian duct cysts and rarely extends above the base of the prostate and is confined to the prostatic boundary. They are symptomatic only when they are large enough to compress the ejaculatory ducts. Müllerian duct cysts are formed due to failure of regression of Müllerian ducts causing saccular dilatation. These cysts are located around the verumontanum and extend beyond the prostate.[17]

Seminal vesicle cysts: It can be congenital or acquired, presenting with recurrent infections. These are thin-walled cysts located in relation to postero-lateral aspect of urinary bladder. They can protrude into the bladder mimicking an ureterocoele. Since these cysts communicate with seminal vesicles, its lumen contains spermatozoa. It is very often associated with ADPKD which can have bilateral seminal vesicle cysts.[17]

Congenital bilateral absence of vas deferens: It is mainly due to the agenesis/aplasia of vas deferens. One of the most common causes is cystic fibrosis and the USG findings show hypoplastic seminal vesicles and ejaculatory ducts with an epididymal remnant composed of a firm and distended caput region along with agenesis of vas deferens.[18]

MISCELLANEOUS CONDITIONS THAT CAUSE INFERTILITY

Erectile dysfunction: It can be due to organic or psychological causes. The organic causes can be vascular, endothelial, myogenic, neurologic, local structural and endocrine disorders. However, vascular insufficiency is seen in majority of cases. The main objective of imaging is to distinguish between vascular and nonvascular causes. Penile Doppler is done only in cases where phosphodiesterase 5 inhibitors do not have any effect. Penile Doppler is done by first giving intra-cavernosal injection of prostaglandin E1 followed by examination of cavernosal arteries and response to spectral waveforms. These waveforms are sampled in repeated 5 minutes intervals until maximum systolic velocity (greater than 35 cm/sec) and minimum diastolic velocity (negative value or close to 0 cm/sec) is reached. Peak systolic velocity less than 25 cm/sec suggests severe arterial disease. Dampened waveforms and high velocity jets suggest proximal arterial stenosis. Standard grey scale USG can be used to detect nonvascular causes like plaques, fibrosis, peyronie's disease and other conditions.[19,20]

Ejaculatory dysfunction: The main causes are: (a) Premature ejaculation, (b) Anorgasmia (inability to achieve orgasm), (c) retrograde ejaculation (semen goes back into male's bladder), (d) Anejaculation (inability to ejaculate).[21]

SUMMARY

A detailed work up of the male partner using a set protocol as defined above to reach the crux of the problem. Imaging has a key role to understand the cause of infertility and therefore direct necessary timely action by differentiating obstructive from non-obstructive causes.

REFERENCES

1. Pardeep K Mittal, Brent Little, Peter A Harri, Frank H Miller, Lauren F Alexander, Bobby Kalb, Juan C Camacho, Viraj Master, Matthew Hartman, Courtney C. Moreno. Radio Graphics Role of Imaging in the Evaluation of Male Infertility 2017;37(3):837–54.
2. Cooper TG, Noonan E, von Eckardstein S, et al. World Health Organization reference values for human semen characteristics.
3. Ammar T, Sidhu PS, Wilkins CJ. Male infertility: the role of imaging in diagnosis and management.
4. Krausz C. Male infertility: pathogenesis and clinical diagnosis.
5. Franco B, Guioli S, Pragliola A et al. A gene deleted in Kallmann's syndrome shares homology with neural cell adhesion and axonal pathfinding molecules.
6. Ciccarelli A, Daly AF, Beckers A. The epidemiology of prolactinomas.
7. Pilatz A, Altinkilic B, Köhler E, Marconi M, Weidner W. Color Doppler ultrasound imaging in varicoceles: Is the venous diameter sufficient for predicting clinical and subclinical varicocele?
8. Browne RF, Geoghegan T, Ahmed I, Torreggiani WC. Intratesticular varicocele.

9. Cross JJ, Berman LH, Elliott PG, Irving S. Scrotal trauma: a cause of testicular atrophy.

10. Cuckow PM, Frank JD. Torsion of the testis.

11. Dohle GR. Inflammatory-associated obstructions of the male reproductive tract.

12. Backus ML, Mack LA, Middleton WD, King BF, Winter TC 3rd, True LD. Testicular microlithiasis: imaging appearances and pathologic correlation.

13. Fawzy F, Hussein A, Eid MM, El Kashash AM, Salem HK. Cryptorchidism and fertility. Clin Med Insights Reprod Health

14. Coursey Moreno C, Small WC, Camacho JC, et al. Testicular tumors: what radiologists need to know—differential diagnosis, staging, and management.

15. Wosnitzer MS, Goldstein M. Obstructive azoospermia.

16. McQuaid JW, Tanrikut C. Ejaculatory duct obstruction: current diagnosis and treatment.

17. Shebel HM, Farg HM, Kolokythas O, El-Diasty T. Cysts of the lower male genitourinary tract: embryologic and anatomic considerations and differential diagnosis.

18. Dörk T, Dworniczak B, Aulehla-Scholz C et al. Distinct spectrum of CFTR gene mutations in congenital absence of vas deferens.

19. Patel DV, Halls J, Patel U. Investigation of erectile dysfunction.

20. Fitzgerald SW, Erickson SJ, Foley WD, Lipchik EO, Lawson TL. Color Doppler sonography in the evaluation of erectile dysfunction: patterns of temporal response to papaverine.

21. Sigman M. Introduction: Ejaculatory problems and male infertility.

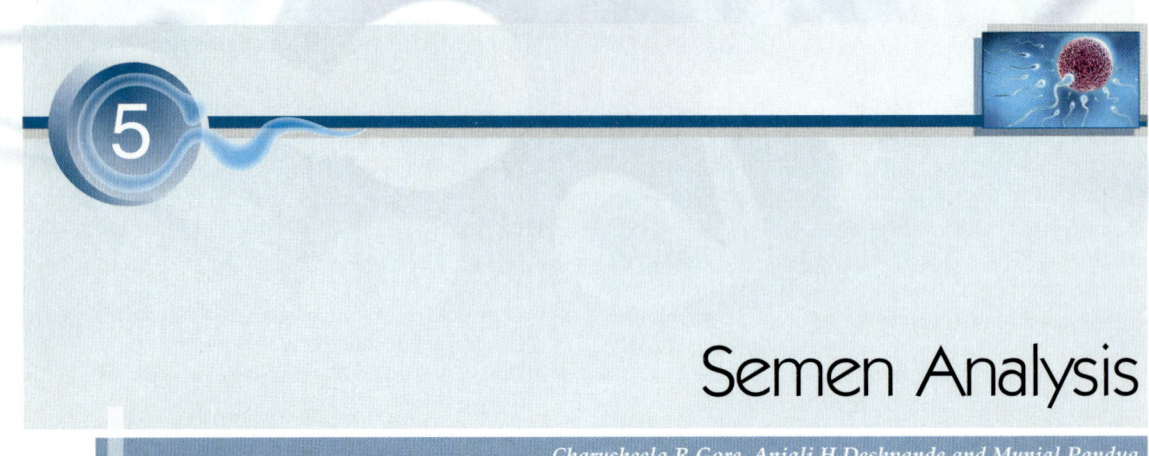

Charusheela R Gore, Anjali H Deshpande and Munjal Pandya

Semen Analysis

Though India is world's second most populated country, the problem of decline in fertility rate has been reported. According to Indian Society of Assisted Reproduction, infertility currently affects 10–14% of Indian population, affecting about 27.5 million couples. Total fertility rate has fallen from 4.97 in 1975-80 to 2.3 in 2015–20. National Family Health Servey 4, also indicated sharp fall in fertility rate among urban Indian population.

When it comes to identifying the causes, 30% times it is attributed to male partner and female partner each, while 30% times to both partners and 10% times it is idiopathic.

A systematic investigative approach is very essential in these couples. Semen analysis is the basic, first line and very important test to assess male fertility. It is a panel of tests which evaluates male reproductive organs and glands. Abnormal results in these test parameters points towards male factor infertility and necessity of further hormonal and clinical assessment.

As semen analysis remains the first and commonly used tests in males, it should be performed meticulously with proper quality control. The recent WHO guidelines given in 5th edition which is published in 2010 are very important in this regard. There are certain changes in reference values in this edition as compared to 4th edition which was published in 1999.

Sample Collection

There should be a standard protocol to be followed during semen analysis which starts from the sample collection itself.

The period of sexual abstinence is very important. It should be between 2–7 days. Usually it is kept 3 days by most of the laboratories. Shorter period may give low sperm count. The motility may get affected due to longer abstinence. If additional sample has to be taken, period of abstinence should be kept constant.

Clear instructions should be given to the patient before obtaining the sample. It should be collected preferably in the private room attached to the lab by masturbation. The sample should be obtained in a clean, wide mouth glass/nontoxic plastic container.

If patient is unable to produce sample in lab, home collection can be done. Ejaculation after coitus interruptus may lead to loss of first portion of ejaculate which is rich in sperms, making this method unreliable. So clear instructions of collection of entire ejaculate should be given.

If condoms are used, they must be free of spermicide agents and nontoxic, otherwise it will interfere with sperm motility.

The sample collected outside should be kept and transported to lab between 20 and 37° C temperature.

Macroscopic Examination/ Physical Examination

It includes assessment for quantity/volume, colour, liquefaction time, viscosity, odour, etc. It should start within 30 mins of collection but never after an hour as dehydration changes or temperature may affect it.

Immediately after collection the semen is semisolid and coagulated. It starts liquefying and it looks homogenous grey-opalescent later.

Appearance

Clear, translucent sample may be azoospermic or oligospermic. Red brown colour may indicate infection or blood. Yellow colour may be due to long abstinence or infections, drugs, etc.

Volume

Minimum Volume should be 1.5 ml. It can be up to 6 ml. Low volume can be due to incomplete collection, stress during collection or secretory dysfunction of accessory glands.

Viscosity

If we drop semen sample through a wide bore plastic pipette, it will form discrete drops. If there is thread formation >2 cm, it is abnormal.

Viscosity can be reduced by gently passing sample through large bore needle or by treatment with chymotrypsin.

Odour

Very strong odour indicates infection.

Liquifaction

The semen which is initially a coagulated semisolid mass in fresh condition, begins to become thinner, i.e liquefy which initially looks heterogeneous and later becomes watery, homogenous. This is due to proteolytic enzymes present in prostatic fluid. Usual time taken is 15 mins at room temperature or at 37°C.

If sample liquefies after 30 mins, it is delayed liquefaction and incomplete if at 60 mins or not liquified. Liquifaction in such samples can be induced by addition of physiologic media. Liquefaction is assessed by both gross and microscopic examination.

Biochemical Analysis

pH: The pH is dependent on acidic prostatic secretions and alkaline seminal fluid. The lower reference value is 7.2 (range 7.2–8).

A more acidic pH (<7) would indicate contamination of sample, blockage of ejaculatory ducts, congenital bilateral absence of vas deference or partial retrograde ejaculation. A more alkaline pH (>8) would indicate presence of infective pathology.

Fructose: It is indicator of seminal vesicle function. Very low fructose, semen volume and pH indicates obstructive pathology, i.e. its absence in semen. Post-ejaculate urine analysis can be done to rule out retrograde ejaculation.

Microscopic Examination

It includes observation of sperm agglutination, aggregation, other cells (leucocytes, epithelial cells, debris), assessment of sperm motility, sperm concentration, total sperm count, sperm morphology and viability.

Aggregation and Agglutination of Sperms

Adherence of immobile spermatozoa to each other or motile spermatozoa to mucous, epithelial or nonepithelial cells is nonspecific aggregation.

When motile sperms stick to each other either head to head, tail to tail or mixed, it is called agglutination. If significant, it warrants antisperm antibody testing.

Round Cells and Cell Debris

These should be counted and different stains can be applied to identify leucocytes from immature germ cells. Leucocytes $>1 \times 10^6$

WBC/ml is abnormal. Increased debris is also abnormal sign and may indicate infection.

Sperm Motility

By taking a small drop of well mixed sample and observing it under microscope at 40X will give an idea about the motility. It should be done after the semen gets liquefied, usually at 30–40 mins. after collection, but within one hour. Minimum 200 spermatozoa should be assessed for motility. It is graded as progressive or nonprogressive and immotile.

Progressive motility (PR): Spermatozoa moving actively (linear or in large circle), regardless of speed.

Nonprogressive motility (NP): Any other pattern of motility but with an absence of progression.

Immotile (IM): No movement.

One has to specify total motility (PR + NP) and among the motile group, progressive motility. The lower reference limit for total motility (PR + NP) is 40% and for progressive motility m (PR) is 32%.

Total number of PR sperms in the ejaculate are obtained by:

Total motile sperm count (PR) = Total number of spermatozoa in ejaculate × percentage (%) of progressively motile sperms

Reduced motility can be due to infection in prostate or seminal vesicles.

Absent motility could be due to antisperm antibodies or Kartagener's syndrome.

Sperm Numbers and Sperm Concentration

It is done after liquefaction of the sample. It can be done in improved Neubauer chamber or Makler chamber (Figs 5.1 and 5.2).

Lower reference limit for sperm concentration is 15×10^6 spermatozoa/ml.

Total sperm count and sperm concentration are not synonymous. Total sperm count refers to number of spermatozoa in entire ejaculate.

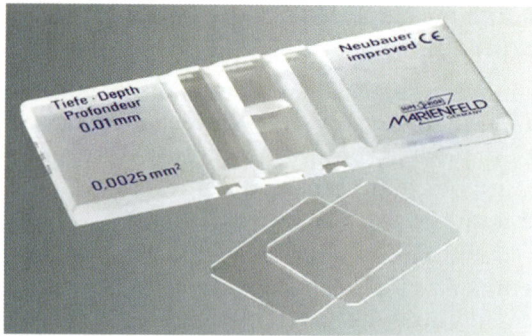

Fig. 5.1: Improved Neubauer chamber.

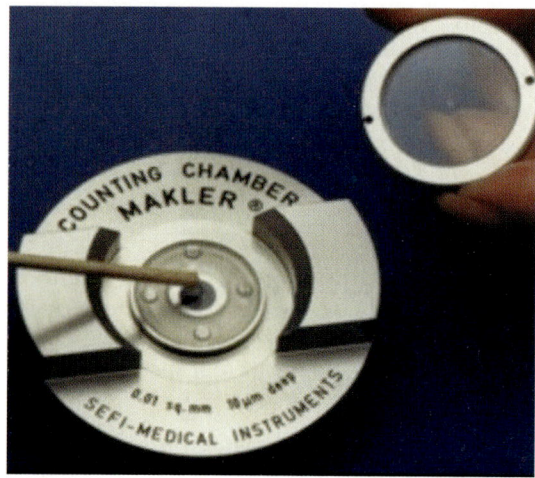

Fig. 5.2: Makler chamber.

Total sperm count = Sperm concentration × semen volume.

The lower reference limit is 39×10^6 spermatozoa/ejaculate.

Sperm morphology

It is very important parameter but is very complex and there is a lot of interobserver variation in reporting.

To observe the morphology, smears are prepared from semen and stained with PAP, Eosin Nigrosin, H&E stain, etc. The smear is examined under oil immersion lens and percentage of abnormal/normal sperms is calculated (Figs 5.3 and 5.4).

The location of abnormality is noted. It can be in head, neck, middle piece or tail.

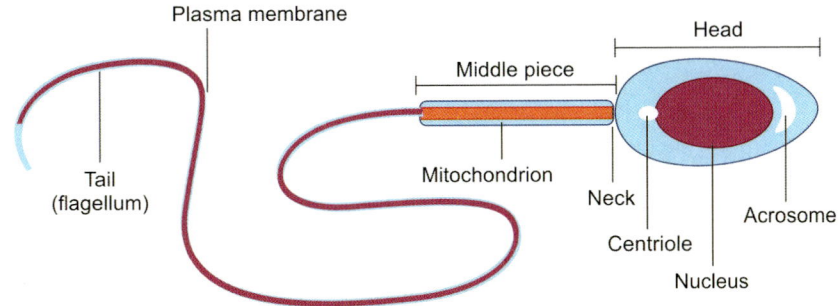

Fig. 5.3: Morphology of normal sperm.

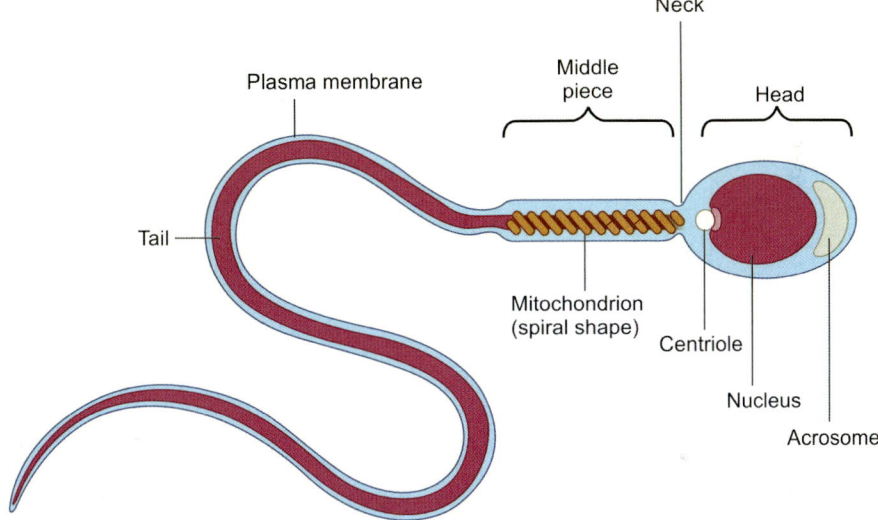

Fig. 5.4: Morphology of abnormal sperms.

The variation from normal should be noted (Fig. 5.4).

Head defects could be large, small, tapering, pyriform, double, round head, etc.

In middle piece, there could be thinning, bent neck, thick irregular midpiece, cytoplasmic droplets, etc.

In the tail, there could be double tail, coiled tail, stumpy tail, multiple tails, etc.

Lower reference limit for normal forms is 4%.

Sperm Vitality

It is done after sample is liquefied, usually at 30 mins. It is measured by assessing the membrane integrity of the cell. It has importance when less than 40% spermatozoa show progressive motility. It can be assessed by dye exclusion or hypotonic swelling. The dead sperms will have damaged membrane and will take up the dye. The viable sperms will swell in hypoosmotic solutions.

The stains used are eosin Y, nigrosin, etc.

Lower reference limit for vitality is 58%.

Evaluation of Antisperm Antibodies (ASA)

If spermatozoa shows agglutination in wet smears, there could be presence of antibodies, though their role is controversial. There are two immunoglobulin classes, IgA, IgG.

IgM, due to large size, are rarely found. There are direct tests and indirect tests. The direct tests are:

- Mixed antiglobulin reaction (MAR) test and Immunobead (IB) test. These detect Ab on spermatozoa.
- The indirect tests detect ASA in seminal plasma, blood or cervical mucus. If the number of motile spermatozoa is less, the indirect tests can be used.
- When the ASA tests are positive (50% or more As Ab binding) additional tests of sperm—cervical mucus penetration should be performed.

Other Biochemical Tests

- Total zinc, total acid phosphatase, total citric acid (prostatic marker).
- Alpha glucosidase, carnitine (epididymis marker).

Computer Aided Semen Analysis (CASA)

This was introduced in 1985. As semen analysis is a complex set of tests, it is difficult to computerize it completely. It mainly assesses the sperm movements. Individual sperm is traced for the speed and trajectory, which can be used as important factor for sperm's ability. Differentiation of spermatozoa from other similar cells and debris is difficult in automation. However, recent advances in technology, particularly with the use of fluorescent DNA stains and tail-detection algorithms, now allows sperm concentration and motility assessment. Image analysis technique has also made it possible to perform computer-aided sperm morphometric assessment.

Many clinical laboratories are not opting for automation due to the disparity in cost of the equipment and workload, as well as manual examination back up, to consolidate the results.

Post-coital test (Sims Huhner test): Mainly done to rule out cervical factor, this test focuses on interaction between sperm and cervical mucus at the time of ovulation. Intercourse is avoided for at least two days before the test. Just when the follicle is mature and about to ovulate, couple is advised to have intercourse. They need to visit laboratory around 6–10 hours after the intercourse. Cervical mucus is taken from endocervix and examined under microscope. Actively motile sperm with forward motion in a thin watery mucus is considered to be adequate test result and rules out cervical factor of infertility. If test does not yield satisfactory results, next test can be done after 2–3 hours of intercourse, but early testing may have many sperm with potential shorter life span, giving false sense of adequacy. Immobilized sperm with side to side shaking suggests antisperm antibodies on sperm or in cervical mucus.

DNA Fragmentation Test

Deoxyribonucleic acid or DNA is the genetic material that contains instructions for embryo to develop and survive.

Each DNA molecule has two strands and four bases which act as building blocks and always follow the same order or sequence. When one or more strands are broken, it can lead to infertility and compromise the health of embryo.

Sperm DNA damage testing has strong association with early fertility checkpoint. These include: fertilization, reduced implantation, miscarriage.

Four tests most commonly used today are:

1. SCSA—Sperm Chromatin Structure Assay
2. TUNEL—Terminal Transferase dUTP Nick End Labelling Assay
3. Sperm chromatin Dispersion SCD or Hallow Test
4. Comet Assay

Sperm Chromatin Structure Assay

SCSA is fluorescence cell sorter test which measures the susceptibility of sperm DNA to denaturation after exposure to heat and acid.

TUNEL Assay

TUNEL assay detects nicks, i.e. free end of DNA by incorporating fluorescently stained nuclides.

Cells can be assessed either microscopically or by flow cytometry, i.e. FCM analysis.

By viability stain, DNA damage is measured in life sperms which has prevented inaccuracy of previous method of measuring damage in the dead sperms also.

Sperm Chromatin Dispersion Test–Halo Test

This is a simple and inexpensive assay, it measures absence of damage rather than damaged DNA in the sperm.

Comet Assay

Second generation sperm DNA test, it quantifies the actual amount of DNA fragments streamed out from the head of unbroken DNA. They resemble a heavenly comet tail, hence the name. The comet is sensitive, repeatable and capable of detecting damage of every sperm.

Unexplained infertility is no more unexplained. 80% of idiopathic infertility have sperm damage more than 25%. This suggests that sperm DNA damage is the cause of infertility in substantial number.

Offering IVF and IUI with such damage can lead to treatment with low chances of success.

So, if DNA fragmentation test is incorporated in routine clinical cases, we could direct these patients directly to ICSI (Intra Cytoplasmic Sperm Injection), avoiding IVF and IUI with repeat failures and heartache.

DNA Fragmentation Index—DFI

- (% of DFI = % sperm cells containing damaged DNA)
- <15% DFI α Excellent to good sperm DNA integrity

- >15 to ≤ 25% DFI α Good to fair sperm DNA integrity
- >25 to <50% DFI α Fair to poor sperm DNA integrity
- >50% DFI α Very poor sperm DNA integrity
- Various studies carried out shows <25% DFI had live births of 33% following IVF treatment and
- >50% DFI had much lower live birth rate– 13%.

THE HYPO-OSMOTIC SWELLING TEST

The hypo-osmotic swelling test (HOS) evaluates the functional integrity of sperms, plasma membrane and also serves as useful indicator of fertility potential of sperm. The influx of fluid due to hypo-osmotic stress causes the sperm tail to coil and balloon or swell. The higher percentage of swollen sperms indicates the presence of sperm having functional and intact plasma membrane.

The HOS test is performed by combining 0.1 ml of ejaculate with 1 ml of hypo-osmotic solution by mixing 7.35 gm sodium citrate and 13.51 gm of fructose in 1 litre of distilled water. Wait for 30 to 60 minutes at 37 °C. 100 to 200 spermatozoa are observed on phase contrast microscopy, percentage of spermatozoa with tail changes (swollen HOS positive spermatozoa) is determined, spermatozoa can be fixed by adding formalin after incubation period.

Normal if ejaculate contains 60% or more HOS positive spermatozoa, 50 to 59% considered as gray zone and such cases can be assigned for IVF.

Optional Tests

- Reactive oxygen species
- Human sperm–oocyte interaction tests
- Human zonapellucida binding tests
- Assessment of the acrosome reaction
- Zona-free hamster oocyte penetration test
- Assessment of sperm chromatin

BIBLIOGRAPHY

1. World Health Organization. WHO laboratory manual for the examination and processing of human semen. 5th ed. Geneva: 2010.

2. Sikka SC, Hellstrom WJG. Current updates on laboratory techniques for the diagnosis of male reproductive failure. Asian Journal of Andrology 2016;18:392–401.2010. doi: 10.4103/1008-682X.179161; published online: 8 April 2016.

3. Fredricsson B, Björk G. Morphology of postcoital spermatozoa in the cervical secretion and its clinical significance. Fertil Steril 1977;28:841–845.

4. Kawthalkar SM. Semen analysis in: Essentials of Clinical Pathology. New Delhi: Jaypee Brothers Medical Publishers(P)Ltd;2010;159–166.

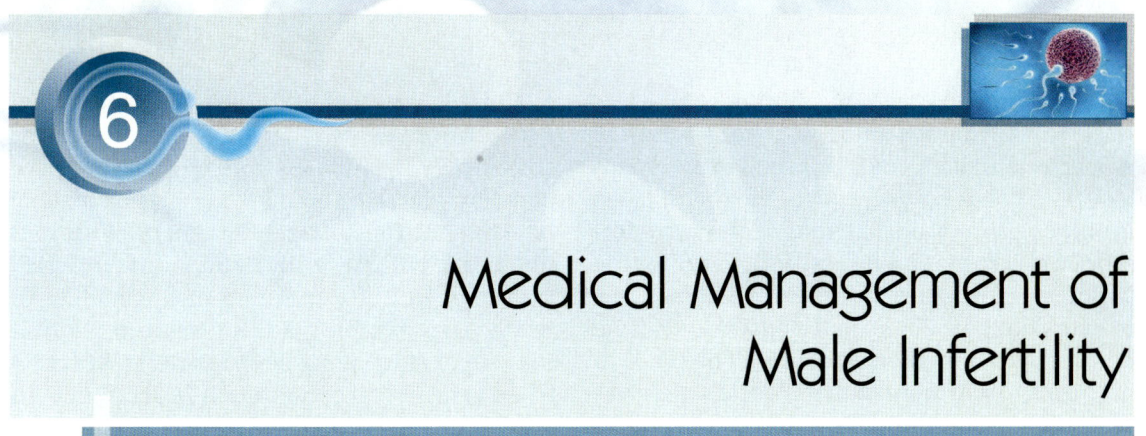

Medical Management of Male Infertility

Anand K Shinde

Male factor infertility amounts to almost 50% workload in an infertility unit and about 75% workload in Andrology unit, the remaining 25% being sex related and STDs or oncology or lower urinary tract related cases. Medical Management of male infertility helps in two ways, one it helps control costs in some cases by reducing dependence on Assisted Reproduction Technology (ART),[1] secondly it gives us opportunities to improve general health of the infertile man in more than one way.[2–4] Pre-ejaculation improvement in semen is the aim of medical management in these cases. Medical therapies alone or in combination with surgery and ART is an essential part of infertility practice. Take an extreme example of the man diagnosed as Non Obstructive Azoospermia (NOA). Here it is wise to see if prior medical treatment will help subsequent surgical retrieval of sperms for wife's ICSI procedure.[5] This type of optimization by medical management is possible in many aetiologies as outlined in this chapter.

The so called 'normal semen profile' is outlined by WHO, 5th edition of *Manual for Semen Analysis*. For semen to be 'normal' the man should have no addictions, should be young, free from male accessory gland infections (MAGI), should have testes in the scrotum (descent), free from any 'heat stress', with normal testicular volume and elasticity (indicating presence of good number of functioning seminiferous tubules), no scrotal pathology (tumor, inflammation, varicocele, hydrocele, etc.) on clinical or ultrasound examination, good output from both semini-ferous compartment (mature sperms) and Leydig's cells (local and circulating testo-sterone) with normal endocrine profile, normal genetic profile, good balance between Reactive Oxygen Species (ROS) production and Total Anti-oxidant Capacity (TAC) in semen, sperms formed in good number and formed well as morphological view goes, free from sperm aneuploidy and low % of sperms with DNA fragmentation, also having normal subcellular organelle and motion kinetics, vitality, capacitation and fertilizing ability. Also required are healthy excurrent trans-portation from testes to penile urethra, normal seminal plasma volume, viscosity, pH, proteo-mics, absence of leukocytes in the semen and finally all the good semen must be efficiently and repeatedly delivered into upper vagina near cervix of wife! One can keep researching into what may go wrong in all above factors and which medical intervention will help enhance his fertility. Take example of the paradox of maintaining blood–testis barrier to protect sperms from autoimmunity and at the same time protect the glands and testes from ascending uro-pathogens.[6] The pheno-menon is quite complex to understand, but in that lies the beauty of medical research helping andrological issues!

Because this chapter has limited space it is wise to outline only areas where medical management works or is reported to work and to open readers' minds to the principles involved in arriving at diagnosis and subsequent therapy and its results. Knowing the difference between curable/treatable and irreversible pathologic aetiologies saves time and costs for the infertile couple. The place of empirical treatment will be touched upon when necessary. Some drug usage can be off-label.[7] So issues involved in off-label drug usage are to be understood by the andrologist and the client should be counselled accordingly.

There are some obvious areas where medical interventions may help. Such examples are:

1. Hypogonadotrophic Hypogonadism (HH) especially post-pubertal HH
2. Excessive Reactive Oxygen species which cause sperm plasma membrane damage and sperm DNA fragmentation
3. Factors inducing apoptotic pathways in germ cells and spermatozoa
4. Androgen deficiency states
5. Male accessory gland infections (MAGI)
6. Erectile and ejaculation dysfunctions
7. Pre- and Post-chemo radiation to brain, abdomen, scrotal malignancies
8. Obesity and metabolic syndrome
9. Varicocele
10. Non-Obstructive Azoospermia (NOA)
11. Idiopathic oligo asthenospermia
12. Hyperprolactinemia, etc.

The easiest to understand but uncommon to find in practice is the treatable cause, viz. HH or hypogonadotrophic hypogonadism where S. FSH, S. LH, S. Testosterone are low or near lower normal level and semen parameters are deranged with symptoms of hypoandrogenism. And while the aetiology of HH may be treatable or not treatable, semen production and androgen output can improve with medications when testicular size is post-pubertal.[8] HH can be secondary to pathology involving hypothalamus and pituitary like Kallman's syndrome, Prader-Willi syndrome, Prolactinomas, other tumors, infections or sometimes it is idiopathic. In cases of HH, clinicians have to be alert about any history of exogenous testosterone or anabolic steroid intake by patient, with or without prescription, e.g. in body builders and athletes. In these cases stopping androgens and waiting to recover from azoospermia or oligospermia is advisable.[9] To hasten the recovery of spermatogenesis inj. hCG or oral clomiphene citrate (CC) have been used. In classic HH one needs to replace the gonadotropins which are low.[10] Main constraints are monetary as the treatment with HCG, HMG, rFSH can take months or years for restoring spermatogenesis and sperms to appear in the ejaculate. In some cases it may not resume if testes are small or undescended (cryptorchidism). In HH usually the androgen levels rise quicker than spermatogenesis resumption. One has to guard against supraphysiologic testosterone levels during HCG therapy. If HCG alone in doses 2500 units twice a week is working, more costly HMG injections can be avoided. But after a few months of hCG alone, if no sperms appear,[11] HMG can be added in doses of 150 units IM on alternate days (3 times per week) in addition to HCG. Married life should continue and pregnancies do occur with sperm counts as low as 5 million/mL in young couples with regular coital activity and healthy wife.

Is there a role for gonadotropins when testes themselves are not 'normal' like in hypergonadotrophic situations (raised FSH)? It is noted that in hypergonadotrophic situations,[12] 50% cases show hypoandrogenism (T <300 ng/dL). Any exogenous testosterone supplement simply suppresses the spermatogenic potential and acts rather like male contraceptive. So can we give hCG or HMG or clomiphene in these hypoandrogenic cases? Yes, it may help by correcting hypoandrogenism and more importantly improving the intra-testicular testosterone (ITT) by stimulating the Leydig cells. Normally ITT levels are roughly 100 times more than serum testosterone. Restored ITT levels start the mitotic activity in the spermatogonia and spermatogenesis can resume.[13] That is, the logic behind 'pre-treatment' in cases of NOA (usually a hypergonadotrophic state) before posting them for surgical sperm retrieval. Prior medical treatment improves prognosis of TESE (testicular sperm extraction). Likewise in idiopathic oligoasthenospermia when gonadotrophins are in 'normal' zones can we still try clomiphene citrate (CC) or aromatase inhibitors (AI)? The answer is Yes. After counselling the client that it may not work in a given case and it may have some side effects, but it is worth trying. How do we choose CC or AI or both (CC+AI) in a given case? It is observed that if serum testosterone (T) is lower than 300 ng /dL then CC can be given 25 mg daily orally with periodic monitoring of T levels.[14] If T levels are not in mid-zone (500–600 ng/dL), one may increase the dose to 50 mg CC/day. It is important to see if estradiol (E) levels also rise with rise in T levels resulting in gynaecomastia in the hypoandrogenic males. Aromatase exists in brain, peripheral and central fat and in testes also which converts androgens to estrogen. If T/E ratio is less than 10, then aromatase inhibitors have a role.[15] Dose of anastrozole can be 1 mg orally, alternate days (three times per week) or Letrozole 2.5 mg once a week to 2.5 mg three times a week. With letrozole there is a need to monitor T levels which can shoot above normal. CC and AI can be combined as per T and T/E values, cautiously. Usually positive results on spermatogenesis are observed by 3 months to 6 months. The aim is to achieve natural conception or undertake IUI (intra-uterine insemination). There is no special benefit of these therapies in the obese group. In obesity weight loss, modifying lifestyle, improving insulin resistance help reduce SHBG levels and the free testosterone levels improve. So, above interventions along with correction of T/E ratio is rationally recommended for overweight and obese men with poor spermatogenesis due to deranged metabolism and hypogonadism. It is observed that CoQ levels are lower with debilitating illnesses and endocrine disorders. Interestingly low T levels are associated with low CoQ levels and rectification of Thyroid/androgen parameters improve CoQ levels.

Along with hormone profile, another factors influencing spermatogenesis (quantity) and sperm function (quality) are environmental estrogenic compounds (xenoestrogens) and endogenous overproduction of Reactive Oxygen Species (ROS).[16] There is a common observation that semen parameters are declining globally and also in Indian males,[17] in parallel with increasing use of pesticides and plastics which are sources of environmental estrogen-like compounds which enter our food chain and water supply. They affect the hypothalamo-pituitary-testis axis and spermatogenesis is disturbed. Interestingly ROS excess is shown to increase beta-inhibin production from Sertoli cells, which directly inhibits spermatogenesis. That is the logic behind papers which show use of CC plus anti-oxidants combination to revive spermatogenesis. Sperms themselves produce ROS through their metabolism and some level of ROS vital for their capacitation and fertilizing ability. But sperms have minimal cytoplasm and thus depend on seminal plasma for anti-oxidants and scavenging of ROS to protect themselves from excess ROS. Dead and defective sperms especially sperms with cytoplasmic droplet (immature sperms), seminal leukocytes, centrifugation process of semen washing methods, cryopreservation of sperms contribute to excess ROS production. ROS causes sperm membrane lipid-peroxidation. That affects sperm motility due to loss of its membrane fluidity. Lipid-peroxidation also prevents sperm's interaction with oolemma at fertilization. ROS damages sperm DNA too. Infertility is the net result of these damages.[18] Naturally there is great interest in oral supplements of various anti-oxidants to improve fertilizing ability by preventing ROS effects on spermatozoa. Very large scale randomized controlled trials in this area are lacking but clinicians may choose low cost and safe anti-oxidants and use them over few months, along with lifestyle modifications for achieving pregnancy. Vitamin C and vitamin E are more supported by good quality studies when literature is searched for antioxidant therapy. Overuse of anything including these two can be detrimental and may cause reductive stress instead of oxidative stress! The effect of ROS excess on sperm DNA fragmentation is another aspect[19] where even if you use IVF/ICSI as a method to circumvent severe male factor infertility, the fertilization rate, cleavage rate and percentage of good embryos, percentage of pregnancies and rate of miscarriage and live birth all suffer due to the DNA damage in the sperm nucleus. Sperm DNA fragmentation when not repairable by the oocyte is source of mutations and aneuploidy in the resultant embryos. The percentage of sperm DNA fragmentation beyond 15% of sperms compromise results of any modality of ART and beyond 30% render natural conception or IUI totally unsuccessful. Also the sources of ROS as mentioned above can also cause inappropriate signalling of apoptosis in precursor cell or even in the mature spermatozoa. If apoptotic sperm is picked up for ICSI, the result will be negative.[20] Some correctible factors in avoiding inappropriate apoptotic signalling can be like ensuring good ITT (intratesticular testosterone) levels and avoiding insults like thermal, chemical, chemotherapy or radiation damage to the testes. Neoplastic growths and disturbed apoptosis in seminiferous tubules are related to each other, so after orchidectomy for one-sided testicular tumor, other testis shows poor semen profile.

Presence of leukocytes in semen is another potent source of ROS[21] as well as phogocytosis of sperms. Leukocytes signal the presence of MAGI (male accessory gland infections) or inflammation in testes or conduction pathway. Source for MAGI is rarely hematogenous, it is almost always ascending infection from lower urinary tract.[22] These infections can be shared infections between husband and wife, so wife should also be checked and treated as necessary. Besides routine uro-pathogens, STDs like gonorrhoea and trichomona vaginalis need attention. Some pathogens which are not culturable but are causative for infertility in up to 25% infertile males (and their wives) like chlamydia, mycoplasma, ureaplasma need other tests like polymerase chain reaction (PCR) which are costly.[23] Consequently most clinicians cover leukocytospermia cases with tetracycline or doxycycline and ciproflox or ofloxacin. The length of treatment should be more than two weeks at least for the males with MAGI. Sometimes chronic treatment is necessary. Anti-inflammatory NSAIDs may have a role in a bacterial leukocytospermia (where cultures/PCRs are negative). Besides bacteria, viruses including HPV can cause leukocytospermia, but this aspect of semen study is the most neglected area. HIV and its treatment with anti-retroviral therapies may cause derangement of the semen profile.

Varicocoeles are commonly linked with poor semen profile as a causative entity and surgery is contemplated. Medical intervention by testicular cooling and addition of anti-oxidants orally over 3 to 6 months may show benefit and surgery may be avoided,[24] especially if wife is young and both can wait for effect of medical therapies which are time consuming. Age of the husband was not an issue till recently, but his age is known to cause worsening of oligospermia and increase in DNA fragmentation rate.[25] Also there is age related secondary hypogonadism, in part due to rise in SHBG levels and reduced testosterone levels. Some age related issues are amenable to medical therapies. Erectile dysfunction, without hypertension/diabetes and vascular problems can be very effectively treated with sildenafil or tadalafil oral treatment, after health check up and counselling.

In severe oligospermia as the age advances, azoospermia may occur, so timely sperm cryopreservation for future use is advisable, while continuing treating the couple's infertility.[26]

So far I have not touched the topic of morphology of sperm. During ART there is every effort done to choose normal looking sperm. But for natural conception and for the curiosity of client and treating consultant we need to address this issue of teratospermia. One way of attempting to rectify morphology is to ignore it.[27] He kept aside morphology and concentrated on only TMSC, i.e. total motile sperms count which is product of total sperm count × % of motile sperms. He commented that 'different WHO Classes (O/A/T or their combinations) do not discriminate sufficiently between fertile and infertile male where occurrence of natural conceptions over a fixed duration (3 years) is concerned, after excluding azoospermia. Three groups of TMSC like Gr I TMSC <5 million gives 24% chance of natural conception within three years, Gr II >5 to <20 million TMSC, the chance is 38% in three years and Gr III TMSC >20 million the chance of pregnancy is 56% in three years!

Of course, some types of morphologies are totally incompatible with occurrence of natural conception such as 100% Globozoospermia, 100% 'pin head' sperms, etc; which need different interpretation. In general medical treatments offered for other correctible (non-genetic) teratospermia are the same as for oligo-asthenospermia.

In summary medical management of male infertility aims to reduce costs of treatment by avoiding costly ART procedures or if they are necessary then making ART more successful by prior medical therapy. Cryopreservation of sperms before chemotherapy or radiotherapy for any malignancies is a sensible medical intervention. Hormone manipulations even in severe NOA cases are effective for the eventual success of surgical sperm retrieval. Medical therapies (FSH) can also be tried in less severe cases like idiopathic oligoasthenospermia[28] or even unexplained infertility and couples with apparently 'normal' semen profile but higher DNA fragmentation rates. It has been reported that since advent of ICSI for male factor infertility our attention to medical management has been reduced but this chapter may make you get interested in medical interventions.

REFERENCES

1. Comhair F. Clinical Andrology: From evidence base to Ethics. The 'E' quintet in clinical Andrology, Hum Reprod 2000;15(10):2067–71.
2. Francis ME, et al. The contribution of common medical conditions to erectile dysfunction detection lead to window of curability. J Andrology 2011;32(2).
3. Miner MM, et al. Erectile dysfunction. Does its detection lead to a window of curability? J Andrology 2011;32(2):125–7.
4. Ramranju GA, et al. Association between obesity and sperm quality. Andrologia 2017;e12888.
5. Sandro C, Esteves SC. Clinical management of infertile men with nonobstructive Azoospermia. Asian J Andrology 2015;17:459–70.
6. Hedger M. Immuno-physiology and pathology of inflammation in the testis and epididymis. J Andrology 2011;32:625–40.
7. KOEY, et al. Empirical medical therapy for idiopathic male infertility. J Urol 2012;187:973–80.
8. Warne DW, et al. Predictive factors for spermatogenesis in HH. Fertil Steril 2009;92:594–604.
9. Fronczak C, et al. The insults of illicit drug use on male fertility. J Androl 2012;33:515–28.
10. Gonadotropin Therapy for Infertile Men with Hypogonadotropic Hypogonadism. Journal of Andrology 2007;28(5):644–6.
11. Boulox H G, et al. Induction of spermatogenesis by recombinant FSH in hypogonadotrophic azoospermic man who failed to respond to hCG alone. J Androl 2003;24:604–611.
12. Bober J, et al. High Prevalence of androgen deficiency in NOA. Int J Androl 2012;35:688–94.
13. Shinjo E, et al. Effect of hCG based hormone therapy on intra testicular testosterone levels and spermatogonial DNA Synthesis in men with NOA. Andrology 2013;1:929–35.
14. Katz DJ, et al. Outcomes of Clomiphene Citrate treatment in young hypogonadal men. BJU Int 2012;110: 537–8.

15. Pavlovich CP, et al. Evidence of treatable endocrinopathy in infertile men. J Urol 2001;165: 837–41.

16. Comhaire FH, et al. Combined conventional/ antioxidant "Asthaxanthin" treatment for male infertility: A double blind randomized trial. Asian J Androl 2005;7(3):237–62.

17. Dama MS, et al. Secular Changes in the semen quality in India during past 33 years. J Androl. 2012;33(4):740–5.

18. Gharagozloo P, et al. The role of sperms oxidative stress in male infertility and the significance of oral antioxidant therapy. Human Reproduction 2011;26(7):1628–40.

19. Barroso G, et al. Analysis of DNA fragmentation, plasma membrane translocation of phosphatidylserine and oxidative stress in human spermatozoa. Hum Reproduction 2000;15:1338–44.

20. Greco E. et al. ICSI in cases of sperm DNA damage: beneficial effect of oral anti-oxidant treatment. Hum Reproduction 2005;20(9): 2590–94.

21. Saleh RA, Agarwal A, et al. Lecocytospermia is associated with increased reactive oxygen species production by human spermatozoa. Fertil Steril 2002;78:1215–24.

22. Soffer Y, et al. Male genital mycoplasmas and Chlamydia trachomatis—relationship with accesory gland function, sperm quality and auto-immunity. Fertil Steril 1990;53(2):331–6.

23. Noura A, et al. Prevalence of Chlamydia trachomatis, mycoplasma hominis infections and seminal quality infertile and fertile men in Kuwait J Andrology 2012;33(6):1323–9.

24. Cavallini G, et al. Cinnoxicam and L Carnitine treatment for idiopathic varicocele associated Oligoasthenospermia. J Andrology 2004;25: 761–70.

25. Schmid TE, et al. The effects of male age on sperm DNA damage in healthy non-smokers. Human Reproduction 2002;22(1):180–7.

26. Song SH, et al. Natural coure of severe oligozoospermia in infertile male: Influence on future fertility potential. J of Andrology 2010;31:536–9.

27. Brandes M, et al. Severity of oligo-teratozoospermia no longer determines overall success rate in male subfertility. Int J Andrology 2011;34: 614–23.

28. Colpi GM, et al. European Academy of Andrology guideline for Management of OAT. Andrlogy 2018;6:513–24.

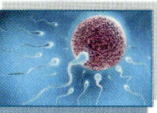

Surgical Management of Male Infertility

Shahaji Chavan, Yogendra Modi and Shrenik Shah

In last decade, diagnostic management strategies of male infertility have undergone tremendous reformations, making male infertility one of the fastest improving fields among all subspecialities in urology. The substantially increased success in the management of male factor infertility witnessed in last few years is due to enhanced techniques in microsurgical reconstruction for obstruction,[1–4] varicocelectomy for enhancement of spermatogenesis,[5, 6] and refined surgical techniques for sperm retrieval[7] along with the successful application of *in vitro* fertilization (IVF) with intracytoplasmic sperm injection (ICSI). Even men with testicular failure once regarded as dismal cases, can now father biological offspring.[8]

In this era of medical advances, with the help of modalities like, IVF and ICSI, it has become possible to make an infertile male capable of conceiving even in most severe forms of irreversible ductal obstructions or even in nonobstructive azoospermia. It is, however, a costly procedure and an intense process for the female partner, with associated risks of complications including ovarian hyperstimulation and multiple gestations, as well as complications of the procedures for oocyte retrieval. Moreover, because it evades all natural biological barriers, ICSI raises realistic concerns about passing genetic abnormalities to offspring.[9, 10] Recent studies indicate that specific treatments for male-

factor infertility (microsurgical reconstruction for obstructive azoospermia and varicocelectomy) remain the safest and most cost-effective ways of managing infertile men, whenever available.[11–14] Thus, proper selection of couples for assisted reproductive technologies and careful genetic counseling is necessary.

The development of high-resolution scrotal and transrectal ultrasound has remarkably enhanced diagnostic capabilities. Ultrasound-guided retrieval of sperm provides diagnostic information and also allows retrieval for IVF with ICSI. Similarly, testicular biopsy to confirm the presence of spermatogenesis was generally reserved for men with normal follicle-stimulating hormone (FSH) levels and testicular volumes, the procedure is indicated in all men with obstructive or nonobstructive azoospermia nowadays. Testicular biopsy has made it possible to retrieve sperm and use them for IVF/ICSI/cryopreservation.

For men with irreparable obstructions and nonobstructive azoospermia caused by testicular failure, surgical sperm retrieval, and assisted fertilization *via* IVF/ICSI are viable management options. The development in various techniques for surgical sperm retrieval from testes, epididymis, or seminal vesicles using percutaneous or open surgical approaches have expanded treatment options for infertile men. In particular, use of the operating microscope to identify the individual seminiferous tubules more likely to contain sperm has improved the success of testicular sperm extraction[15] and minimized associated morbidity.[16]

Microsurgical techniques also have been extended to varicocelectomy. Varicoceles, long known to be associated with male infertility, have now clearly been shown to result in progressive duration-dependent testicular insult.[17–24] On this basis, the scope of benefit has expanded over the years. Previously, microsurgical varicocelectomy was reserved only for men with oligospermia, but now it has been applied to men with nonobstructive azoospermia, which has shown promising results in more than 50% of cases with return of normal spermatogenesis.[5, 25] Whereas surgical varicocele repair was previously reserved for already infertile men, earlier intervention now offers the means to salvage remaining testicular function and also to prevent future infertility. It is now evident that varicocele adversely affects Leydig cell function and lowers serum testosterone levels, thus varicocelectomy might be expected to halt or even partially reverse an otherwise inevitable decline.[26] In some selected men, varicocelectomy is an effective treatment for symptomatic age-related androgen deficiency, a condition that has been named *andropause*.

Surgical treatment of male infertility and scrotal disorders poses minor risk to patients and offers the promise of new and improved quality of life for infertile couples. The techniques are technically demanding and require both intensive microsurgical training and a thorough knowledge of the anatomy and physiology of the male reproductive system.

ANATOMY

The main blood supply to the testis is from the testicular (internal spermatic) artery arising directly from the aorta (Figs 7.1 and 7.2). A second blood supply comes from the artery of the vas deferens (deferential artery), which is derived from the hypogastric (internal iliac) artery or the superior vesical artery (also a branch of the hypogastric). Inferior epigastric artery sends off cremasteric (external spermatic) artery, supplying tunica vaginalis, but also sending some branches to testes. Atrophy and/or azoospermia have resulted from testicular artery ligation both in adults and in children. The epididymis has a rich blood supply. The superior and the medial epididymal arteries are derived from the testicular artery. The vasal (deferential) artery supplies the cauda (inferior pole) of the epididymis. Epididymal blood supply would be adequate till superior epididymal artery remains intact. The vas deferens obtains its blood supply from two sources, both anastomosing with each other. The seminal vesical (abdominal) end of the vas derives its blood supply from the deferential (vasal) artery. The vas deferens has no blood supply from the surrounding cremaster muscle or from any blood vessels from the spermatic cord. Therefore, if the vas gets damaged at two different sites, the intervening segment will be devoid of blood supply, making it fibrosed and nonfunctional. Thus, anastomosis at those two sites will be of no use. 7 to 11 tiny efferent convoluted ducts carry sperm and testicular fluid forming the caput of the epididymis. At that level, they freely anastomose with one another. They all join at the distal caput to form a single epididymal tubule from the caput corpus junction all the way to the vas deferens. The left and right ejaculatory ducts enter the prostatic urethra at the level of the utricle.

TESTICULAR BIOPSY

Testicular biopsy is done in azoospermic men with testis of normal size and consistency, palpable vasa deferentia, and normal FSH levels, and a negative serum antisperm antibody assay to distinguish obstructive from nonobstructive azoospermia. Diagnostic

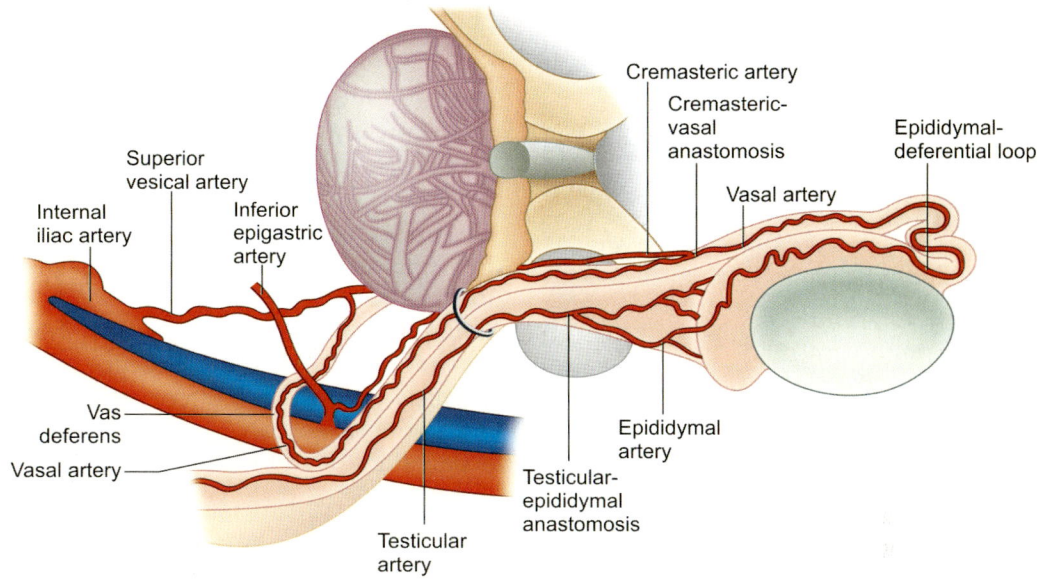

Fig. 7.1: Collateral arterial circulation to the testis.[27]

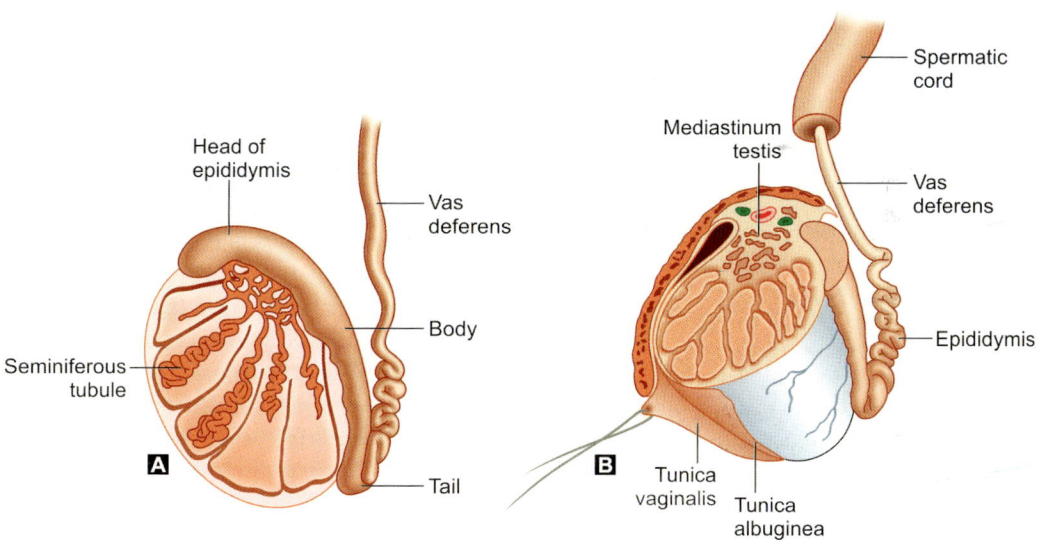

Fig. 7.2: Anatomy of testis.(A) Parts of testis; (B) Cross section of testis.

biopsy is usually performed bilaterally irrespective of the size discrepancy of the two testes. Good spermatogenesis can be sometimes found in small, firm testes, and biopsies of large, healthy testes may reveal maturation arrest (Fig. 7.3).

Open testis biopsy: Microsurgical technique open biopsy remains the gold standard because it provides an optimal amount of tissue both for accurate diagnosis and for retrieval of sperm for IVF. The main goal while performing a testis biopsy is to provide

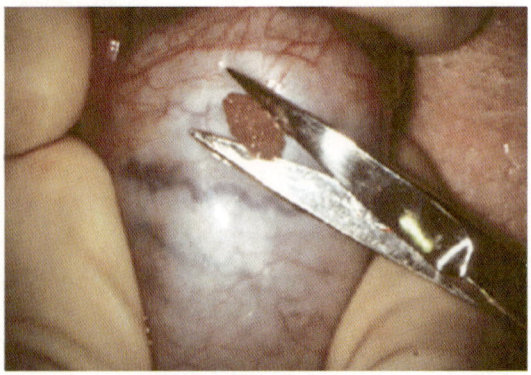

Fig. 7.3: Testicular biopsy/TESE.

an optimal tissue sample, avoid trauma to the specimen, and avoid injury to the epididymis or testicular blood supply. These prerequisites can be met by performing it under magnification (under microscope).

Percutaneous Testis Biopsy

Percutaneous testis biopsy using the same 14-gauge biopsy gun which is used for prostatic biopsy is a blind procedure and could result in unintentional injury to either the epididymis or the testicular artery.

As a therapeutic tool for sperm retrieval, percutaneous biopsy or aspiration is very useful for fresh sperm retrieval for IVF with ICSI in cases of obstructive azoospermia and normal spermatogenesis.

VARICOCELE

Varicocele commonly occurs due to the absence of valves in one of the longest veins of the body, the left gonadic vein that drains in the left renal vein. It is seen in around 15% of the normal males. The rate goes as high as 40% in those with primary infertility and 80% in those having secondary infertility. It is more often bilateral than earlier believed. Progressive deterioration of testicular function is clearly associated with varicocele. Many authors relate the problem to an elevated scrotal temperature due to the lack of heat exchange at the level of the pampini-

form plexus, others describe the toxic effects of elevated venous catecholamines, cortisol and renin.[26] Physical examination can diagnose varicocele, but Doppler sonography must confirm the persistence of a retrograde flow during the Valsalva maneuver.

There are two main indications for the treatment of varicocele: scrotal pain and infertility. A painful varicocele is usually large in size and easily diagnosed but the importance of subclinical varicoceles should be considered even in the presence of a small retrograde flow.[29] A refluent varicocele needs a treatment in case of fertility problem, because the result of the treatment is independent of size of the veins and degree of the retrograde flow.

Both Surgical and nonsurgical techniques for the treatment of a varicocele are available (Fig. 7.4A and B).

- The high ligation technique consists in finding the spermatic vein at the level of the lower pole of the kidney through a retroperitoneal approach. The skin incision is kept horizontally medial to the anterior superior iliac spine, the external oblique muscle is incised, the internal oblique muscle is retracted and the peritoneum is teased away. Vein is easier to be ligated at this juncture. It sometimes happens that some collaterals take their origin from another vein, causing the failure of the procedure in about 2% of the cases. The surgical approach on the right side is more difficult because the right gonadic vein drains in the inferior vena cava.

- Inguinal ligation is done through a low inguinal incision. External oblique aponeurosis is incised, and spermatic cord is isolated. After incising spermatic fascia, dilated veins are identified, ligated and excised. This permits a complete stop in the internal drainage. This technique is safe, but the number of relapses is often high because of difficulties with dissection which leaves patent veins in up to 21% of the cases, unless

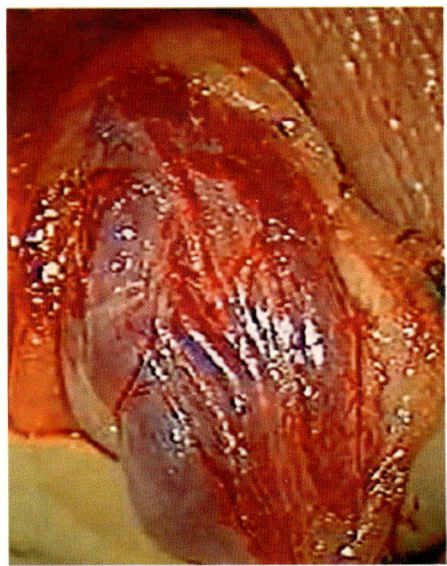

Fig. 7.4A: Microsurgical view of the veins of the pampiniform plexus during varicocele ligation through a subinguinal approach.

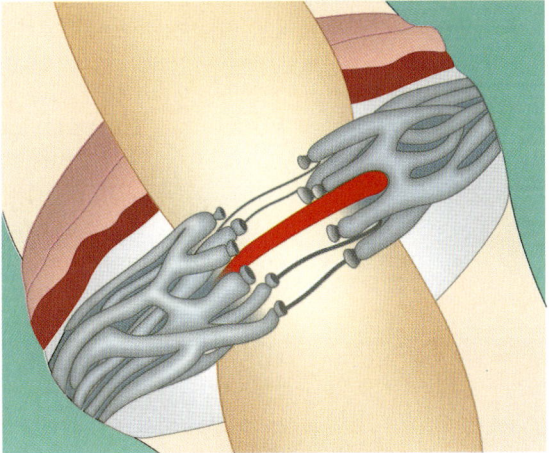

Fig. 7.4B: At the completion of the dissection, only the testicular arteries, cremasteric arteries, lymphatics, and vas deferens with its vessels remain.

it is performed by a skilled surgeon under microscope or magnifying glasses.[28]

• Radiologically controlled embolization is an easy day procedure: After puncture and catheterization of one of the femoral veins, the radiologist identifies the refluant spermatic vein by injecting an iodine dye during a Valsalva maneuver. During maneuver, a sclerotizing solution is injected or a wire coil or a detachable balloon can be placed. This is cost-effective as well as time saving, but it does have a failure rate of around 12% due to anatomical variations in veins. There is also a risk of migration of the sclerotizing agent or coil and it also exposes the patient to irradiation.

• The recent laparoscopic technique has now been extensively used in many centers. After umbilical port is inserted, the peritoneal cavity is insufflated with CO_2 at a pressure of around 14 mm Hg. The vein is easily identified, running under the posterior peritoneum between the sigmoid colon and the internal inguinal ring. Two other ports are inserted, and the pressure is lowered to 8 mm Hg. Titanium clips are used once veins are dissected properly, sparing spermatic artery and the lymphatics. The laparoscopic method is very precise, causes less morbidity with lesser hospital stay (only 24 hours hospitalization) along with reduced recurrences. A skilled laparoscopic surgeon is required in order to avoid the dangers of laparoscopy itself.

Overall results of varicocele repair in collated studies show 50 to 90% improvement in semen quality and 30 to 50% may succeed in getting conceived after 6 to 9 months.[31] For men with azoospermia or severe oligospermia, modest improvement in semen quality after varicocele repair causes a significant impact on a couples' fertility potential.

EJACULATORY DUCT RESECTION

The vas ends in the ejaculatory duct at the level of the verumontanum. Even a small lesion in that region can cause an obstruction, usually bilateral. Such lesion can be inflammatory or can be congenital. It is supposed in case of low semen volume (less than 1.0 ml) and absence of fructose in the seminal plasma. Perineal pain and hematospermia may be accompanying. The rest of the vas deferens is generally normal. Transrectal ultrasound echography is gold standard for diagnosing ejaculatory duct obstruction (Fig. 7.5).

Endoscopy with a resectoscope is done using an incision along verumontanum. Deep resection is sometimes needed and one must be very careful to avoid rectum perforation or sphincter lesion.[30]

VASOVASOSTOMY

Most commonly, obstruction of the vas deferens occurs due to vasectomy. Other uncommon causes are short segmental agenesis, accidental section during hernia repair or postinfectious localized obstruction. Vasovasostomy can be performed anywhere along the scrotal and inguinal part of the vas. It is also theoretically possible intraperitoneally by laparoscopy but generally, as a consequence of vasectomy, it is usually done in the mid or upper part of the scrotum (Figs 7.6A to C).

Modified two-layers technique allows good results: Four 9–0 monofilament absorbable sutures are placed at 6, 9, 3 and 12 o'clock through the serosa and the mucosa in order to approximate the two portions of the vas. Additional four stitches using 9–0 suture are placed in between previous 4 stitches so as to tighten the vas. Microscope is mandatory

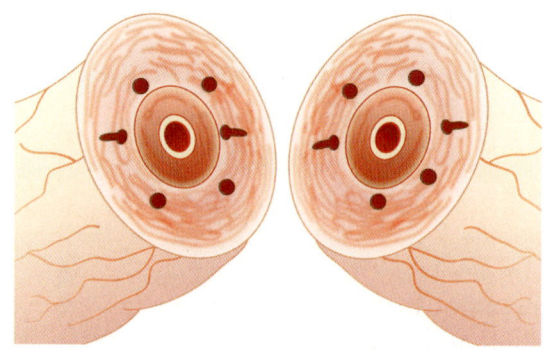

Fig. 7.6A: The abdominal end of the vas is marked in the same way to exactly match the testicular end.

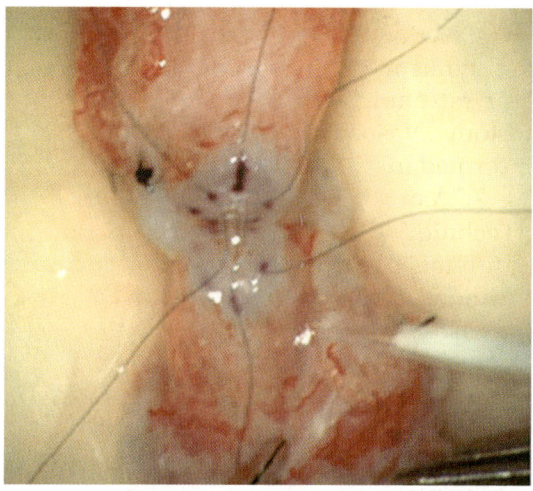

Fig. 7.6B: Sutures passed through the mucosa of the vas.

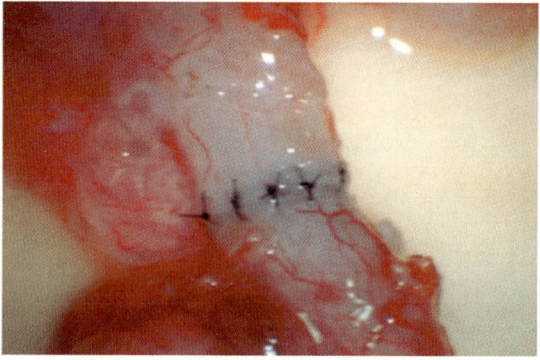

Fig. 7.6C: Outer layer of the vas is approximated.

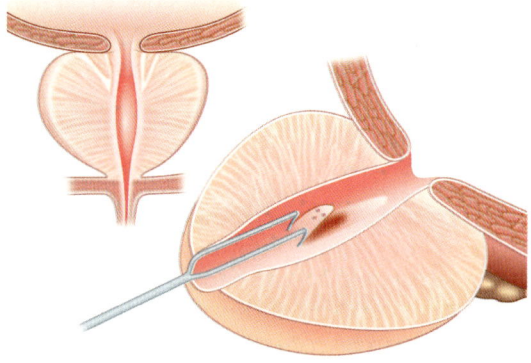

Fig. 7.5: The ejaculatory ducts course between the bladder neck and the verumontanum and exit at the level of and along the lateral aspect of the verumontanum.

for optimal results. In some vasectomy cases a large part of the vas is resected, making tension free direct anastomosis impossible. The epididymis can be dissected free from the testis, being attached only by the head and brought up to the distal end of the vas, thus making anastomosis possible without traction.

It is important to note that the mean time between vasectomy reversal and conception is more than twelve months and, more important, that the fertility rate of the reversal group is the same as in the normal control group.

VASOEPIDIDYMOSTOMY

If obstruction is present at the level of the epididymis in the presence of a normal vas, the first-choice therapy is vasoepididy-mostomy. Vasoepididymostomy shall also be performed in case of unsuccessful vasectomy (Fig. 7.7A and B).

Technique consists of lateral opening of epididymis proximal to the level of obstruc-tion and isolating a single tubule which, later on, is incised, but not transacted, and anasto-mosed side to end.

The results of this procedure show a patency rate of 85% with a pregnancy rate of only 44%. Vasoepididymostomy has a higher pregnancy rate than IVF with ICSI and should be preferred in any case of obstructive sterility at the epididymal level.

ORCHIOPEXY IN ADULTS

This is well known that cryptorchidism is associated with a high incidence of infertility even when unilateral. Spermatogenesis is delicately temperature sensitive. It will also preserve testicular hormonal function. The technique of orchiopexy in adults is similar to that employed for children. Even with a normal contralateral testis, orchiopexy is worthwhile to bring down a unilateral undescended testis to, if possible, a scrotal location where it can be examined. Leydig cell function in undescended testis can be retained. Orchiopexy in adults with bilateral undescended testes can induce spermato-genesis and allow pregnancy. Even a solitary cryptorchid testis, when properly placed in the scrotum, can provide enough testosterone to obviate the need for hormone replacement. When orchiopexy is performed, regular self-examination and yearly sonography are mandatory in adults.

The fate of persistently retractile testis in adults is unknown. These testes may suffer from impaired temperature regulation and impaired spermatogenesis. Scrotal orchiopexy can improve the semen quality and fertility of some of these men. Some men have ectopic testis, in which one testis is behind the other almost in the perineum. This also elevates testis temperature. When scrotal orchiopexy

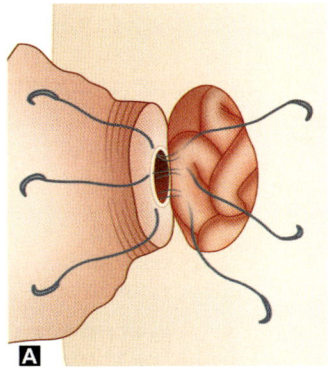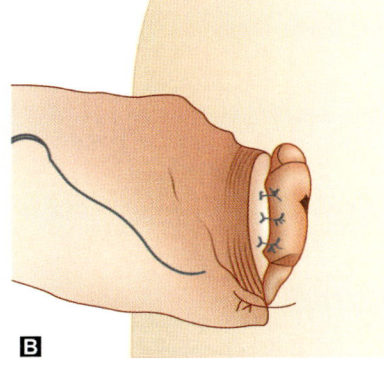

A **B**

Fig. 7.7 A and B: The outer muscularis and adventitia of the vas are then approximated to the cut edge of the epididymal tunica with 6 to 10 additional interrupted sutures of 9–0 nylon double-armed with 100-micron diameter needles.

is performed for retractile or ectopic testis in adults, a dartos pouch operation should be performed. Simple suture orchiopexy of the tunica albuginea of the testis to the dartos, as is performed sometimes to prevent torsion, will not prevent retraction of these testes into the groin. Creation of a dartos pouch will keep the testis well down in the scrotum and permanently prevent retraction. This is also the most reliable and safest technique for the prevention of testicular torsion.

EPIDIDYMAL SPERM ASPIRATION

Bilateral absence or total obstruction of the vas had no cure until recent times. The first description by Temple-Smith of sperm micro-aspiration from the epididymis and *in vitro* fertilization resulting in a pregnancy followed

by Silber who repeated the procedure with success, opened a new field. Silber had better pregnancy rates in cases of agenesis than in those with acquired obstruction. The actual fecundation rate was 70%, with pregnancy rates of 30–50% (Table 7.1).

ICSI WITH TESTICULAR BIOPSY

The most recent development of the intra cytoplasmic sperm injection (ICSI) has opened a new field in making infertile men capable of conceiving, including those with obstructive azoospermia. In other cases, even after a former negative biopsy and elevated FSH, it is usually possible to retrieve living spermatozoa in about 50% of cases.

Biopsy is best performed by exteriorizating both testis and obtaining 3 to 4 small

Table 7.1: Surgical techniques of sperm retrival

	Advantages	Disadvantages
MESA (microsurgical epididymal sperm aspiration	Microsurgical procedure allows lower complication rate. Epididymal sperm has better motitily than testicular sperm. Large number of sperm can be harvested for cryopreservation of multiple vials in a single procedure.	Requires anesthesia and microsurgical skills. Not indicated for nonobstructive azoospermia.
PESA (percutaneous epididymal sperm aspiration)	No microsurgical skill required. Local anesthesia. Epididymal sperm has better motility than testicular sperm.	Complications include hematoma, pain, and vascular injury to testes and obstruction of the epididymis. Variable success in obtaining sperm. Smaller quantity of sperm obtained than with MESA. Not indicated for nonobstructive azoospermia.
TESA (testicular sperm aspiration)	No microsurgical skill required. Local anesthesia. Can be used for obstructive azoospermia.	Immature or immotile testicular sperm. Small quantity of sperm obtained. Poor results in nonobstructive azoospermia. Complications include hematoma, pain, and vascular injury to testes and epididymia.
TESE (testicular sperm extraction)	Low complication rate if performed microsurgically. Perfered technique for nonobstructive azoospermia.	Requires anesthesia and microsurgical skills.

fragments which should be extemporaneously examined in order to find a sperm producing zone in the testis. Percutaneous biopsy has not given good results. More recently it has been suggested to press a slide to the opened testis and look for spermatozoa, under microscope. This technique avoids useless damaging of already small testis. One single spermatozoa can also be picked up from a small testis and can be used for ICSI. This procedure has a comparable fertilization and pregnancy rate.

REFERENCES

1. Matthews GJ, Schlegel PN, Goldstein M. Patency following microsurgical vasoepididymostomy and vasovasostomy: Temporal considerations. J Urol 1995;154(6):2070–3.
2. Chan PTK, Schlegel PN. Vasovasostomia e vaso-epididimostomia Microcirurgicas. In: Neves PA, Netto NR Jr (Eds): Infertilidade Masculina 2002;149–62.
3. Goldstein M, Chan PTK, Li PS. Multi-layer Micro-surgical Vasovasostomy: Tricks of the Trade. Cornell Institute for Reproductive Medicine 2002.
4. Chan PTK, Brandell RA, Goldstein M. Prospective analysis of the post-operative outcomes of microsurgical intussusception vasoepididymostomy. J Urol 2002;167:310.
5. Matthews GJ, Matthews ED, Goldstein M. Induction of spermatogenesis and achievement of pregnancy after microsurgical varicocelectomy in men with azoospermia and severe oligoasthenospermia. Fertil Steril 1998;70:71–5.
6. Chan PTK, Goldstein M. Medical Backgrounder on Varicocele. Drugs of Today 2002;38:59–67.
7. Chan PTK, Schlegel PN. Diagnostic and therapeutic testis biopsy. Curr Urol 2000;1:266–72.
8. Chan PTK, Schlegel PN. Non-obstructive azoospermia. Curr Opinion Urol 2000;10:617–24.
9. Hansen M, Kurinczuk JJ, Bower C, Webb S. The risk of major birth defects after intracytoplasmic sperm injection and *in vitro* fertilization. N Engl J Med 2002;346:725–30.
10. Schieve LA, Meikle SF, Ferre C, et al. Low and very low birth weight in infants conceived with use of assisted reproductive technology. N Engl J Med 2002;346:731–7.
11. Kolettis PN, Thomas AJ. Vasoepididymostomy for vasectomy reversal: A critical assessment in the era of intracytoplasmic sperm injection. J Urol 1997;158:467–70.
12. Pavlovich CP, Schlegel PN. Fertility options after vasectomy: A cost-effectiveness analysis. Fertil Steril 1997;67:133–41.
13. Schlegel PN. Is assisted reproduction the optimal treatment for varicocele-associated male infertility? A cost-effectiveness analysis. Urology 1997;49:83–90.
14. Donovan JF Jr, DiBaise M, Sparks AE, et al. Comparison of microscopic epididymal sperm aspiration and intracytoplasmic sperm injection/ *in vitro* fertilization with repeat microscopic reconstruction following vasectomy: is second attempt vas reversal worth the effort? Hum Reprod 1998;13:387–93.
15. Schlegel PN. Testicular sperm extraction: microdissection improves sperm yield with minimal tissue excision. Hum Reprod 1999;14:131–5.
16. Dardashti K, Williams RH, Goldstein M. Microsurgical testis biopsy: A novel technique for retrieval of testicular tissue. J Urol 2000;163:1206–7.
17. Russell JK. Varicocele, age, and fertility. Lancet 1957;2:222.
18. Lipshultz LI, Corriere JN. Progressive testicular atrophy in the varicocele patient. J Urology. J Urol 1977;117:175–6.
19. Nagler HM, Li X-Z, Lizza EF, et al. Varicocele: Temporal considerations. J Urol 1985;134:411–3.
20. Pathophysiology of varicocele in nonhuman primates: long-term seminal and testicular changes. Harrison RM, Lewis RW, Roberts JA, Fertil Steril 1986,46:500–10.
21. Kass EJ, Chandra RS, Belman AB. Testicular histology in the adolescent with a varicocele. Pediatrics 1989;79:996–8.
22. Hadziselimovic F, Herzog B, Liebundgut B, et al. Testicular and vascular changes in children and adults with varicocele. J Urol 1989,142:583–5.
23. Gorelick J, Goldstein M. Loss of fertility in men with varicocele. Fertil Steril 1993;59:613–6.
24. Sigman M, Jarow JP. Ipsilateral testicular hypotrophy is associated with decreased sperm counts in infertile men with varicoceles. J Urol 1997;158:605–7.
25. Kim ED, Leibman BB, Grinblat DI, et al. Varicocele repair improves semen parameters in azoospermic men with spermatogenic Failure. J Urol 1999;162:737–40.

26. Belker AM, Thomas AJJR, Fuchs EF, Konnak JW, Sharlip ID. Results of 1,469 microsurgical vasectomy reversals by the vasovasostomy study group. J Urol 1991;145:505–11.

27. From Hinman F Jr. Atlas of urosugical anatomy. Philadelphia: Saunders; 1993;497.

28. Biase JN, Nagler MN. The varicocele: current concepts and controversies. Current op the varicocele: current concepts and controversies.

29. Denil J, Jonas U. The management of disturbance of sperm transport. Eur Urol 1992;2:82–7.

30. Hadziselimovic F, Herzog B, Leibundgut B, Jenny P, Buser M. Testicular and vascular changes in children and adults with varicocele. J Urol 1989; 142:583–5.

31. Lipschultz LI, Kessler DL, Monogr. Evaluation and treatment of male infertility. Urol 1986;7.

8

IUI: Prerequisites, Counseling and Informed Consent

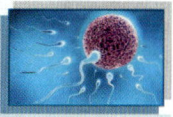

Manish Banker and Neha Sharma

INTRODUCTION

IUI is a therapeutic technique of placing processed sperms via cervix into uterus in order to facilitate fertilization by allowing large number of motile sperms near oocyte. Intrauterine insemination (IUI) with homologous (IUI-H) or donor semen (IUI-D) is frequently used as a first choice of treatment for many infertile couples worldwide.[1]

Treatment by artificial insemination with husband's sperm remains a valuable first choice treatment before starting more invasive and more expensive techniques of assisted reproduction in many cases of human subfertility, especially if tubal patency is proven. It is a simple and noninvasive technique which does not require an expensive infrastructure.

RATIONALE

Rationale behind IUI is that the motile spermatozoa, concentrated in small volume, are placed directly into uterus close to released oocyte. Reason for achieving pregnancy is an increase in the number of motile near the site of fertilization.[2] In addition, this is carried out close to the time of ovulation.

Keeping this in mind, proper diagnosis and pretreatment work-up of the female reproductive tract, proper semen analysis and minimal ovarian stimulation and IUI should be promoted as the first-line treatment in most cases of subfertility.

INDICATION

There are a number of indications for IUI using the husband or partner's semen; these are summarized below.

Indications for Intrauterine Insemination

Effective

1. Male problems leading to problems with deposition of sperms in the vagina: like ejaculatory disturbance, hypospadiasis, impotence.
2. Male subfertility.
3. Cervical factor.
4. Idiopathic/unexplained infertility.

Possibly Effective

1. Immunological infertility.
2. Endometriosis.
3. Ovulatory dysfunction where only ovulation induction has not been successful.

The main indications for donor insemination are:
1. Azoospermia or severe oligoasthenoteratozoospermia where the couple do not wish to undergo IVF.
2. Severe inherited chromosomal disorder in the male partner, Rh incompatibility.

The use of cryopreserved semen in donor insemination programs is now mandatory in most countries, to minimize the possibility of the transmission of human immunodeficiency

virus (HIV) and other infections to the recipients.

CONTRAINDICATION

IUI is contraindicated in women with cervical atresia, cervical mucus hostility, bilateral tubal obstruction, acute genital tract infection and in cases with complete absence of ovulation.

Prerequisites for Insemination (IUI)

Before proceeding to IUI, comprehensive assessment is required. This includes a thorough medical history, clinical examination and appropriate investigations for any possible causes of a couple's infertility.

Insemination should be performed only if the following conditions are met. The minimum requirements for performing the procedure are:

1. Evidence of ovulation
2. At least one patent fallopian tube
3. Adequate numbers of motile sperm
4. Receptive endometrium
5. Absence of documented or suspected active cervical, intrauterine, or pelvic infection.

Evidence of Ovulation

The goal of ovarian stimulation should be the development of a maximum of three dominant follicles. If more than three follicles have developed or two or more mature 15 mm size follicles are seen, insemination should not be undertaken in order to reduce the risk of multiple pregnancies. The chance of a pregnancy was 5% higher when two follicles were stimulated as compared with monofollicular growth and 8% higher when three or four follicles were present. The absolute rate of multiple pregnancies was 0.3% after monofollicular and 2.8% after multifollicular growth.[3]

IUI may be performed in natural cycle as well as in combination with controlled ovarian hyperstimulation (COH). Various drugs used for COH are clomiphene citrate, letrozole, gonadotropin (GN) such as human menopausal gonadotropin (hMG) and/or pure follicle stimulating hormone (FSH). Based on the findings of past research, it has been stated that gonadotropin, either alone or in combination with CC, gives a higher CPR (clinical pregnancy rate) and a lower miscarriage rate following IUI, however, increasing the MPR (multiple pregnancy rate).[4] The higher pregnancy rates after using gonadotropin could be due to a better follicular development, development of multiple follicles and good endometrial thickness. However, gonadotropins are expensive and have certain associated adverse events such as ovarian hyperstimulation syndrome (OHSS), and high-order multiple pregnancies. But, being highly responsive and effective these are used in COH. Using a combination of CC or letrozole and gonadotropin makes COH and IUI more a cost-effective and yet efficient.[5] In women with polycystic ovary syndrome, letrozole appears to be associated with a higher live birth rate, lower rates of multiple pregnancy and lower risk of OHSS than clomiphene citrate.[6]

Ovulation is monitored almost exclusively with ultrasonography. Ultrasound for ovulation induction is usually performed on the third to fifth day of cycle to carry out baseline evaluation, rule out the presence of ovarian or endometrial pathology and to measure antral follicles to determine ovarian reserve. Subsequent monitoring is carried out about a week later and then based on the response.

It is recommended that secondary preventive measures to prevent multiple pregnancies are initiated when three or more follicles ≥ 14 mm are present at the time of HCG injection. These measures include cancelation of the cycle or escape IVF.[7]

A mid-luteal cycle serum progesterone level is tested one week before an expected period (on day 21 of 28 days cycle). Levels >5 ng/ml is consistent with ovulation and no further biochemical assessment is required.

At Least One Patent Fallopian Tube

In order for a woman's reproductive capacity to function correctly, the anatomy and function of fallopian tubes needs to be intact as they play an extremely active role in the process of fertilization. The prevalence of tubal factor infertility varies from 11 to 30% depending on the setting and population. Therefore, the initial investigations of an infertile couple should be confined to assessment of sperm (seminal fluid analysis), pelvic anatomy (transvaginal ultrasound scan), and ovulation and ovarian reserve (follicular phase gonadotrophins, midluteal progesterone). Invasive tubal patency test should be offered after taking into account the overall treatment needs of the couple. So it does not require the routine use of a tubal patency test prior to initiating treatment. The majority of such women who conceive, do so within the first three attempts and only women keen to proceed with further OI or IUI treatment are offered a tubal patency test.[8]

Our current practice is in keeping with data from other studies that confirm a lack of therapeutic and prognostic benefit of routine tubal patency testing prior to initiating IUI in low-risk women.[9] The various options for testing tubal patency are—hysterosalpingogram (HSG), hysterosalpingo-contrast-sonogaphy (HyCoSy) and laparoscopy. HSG could be used as screening test for couples with no prior history of pelvic infection, pervious ectopic pregnancy or endometriosis. HSG has moderate sensitivity of 65% but high specificity (83%) that makes it reliable test for ruling out tubal obstruction. Hysterosalpingography identified bilateral tubal block is found in 24% of couples with secondary infertility with normal sperm and an ovulatory cycle, the figures for those couples with male factor subfertility, or anovulation, are 5% and 7%, respectively. Hysterosalpingo-contrast-sonography is recognized as having greater sensitivity than HSG for detection of intrauterine pathology.[10]

A more comprehensive evaluation of tubal patency can be done by laparoscopy and dye testing. The use of laparoscopy should be limited to cases suspected of having etiologies other than intratubal occlusion such as endometriosis or peritubal adhesion.

Depending upon the factors such as young patient age and lower duration of infertility, IUI can be performed without prior tubal assessment. In summary, a policy of universal invasive tubal patency testing is to be discouraged; instead the investigation and management of tubal factor infertility should be individualized to the needs of patients and populations.

If the tubal patency test shows that only one tube is open, IUI can only be carried out when ovulation is about to occur from the ovary that is on same side. Although there is increased probability of cycle cancellation in patient with single patent tube 34% vs. 5.1% in patient with bilateral patent tubes.[11]

Adequate Number of Motile Sperms

Semen analysis plays a key role in the diagnostics of male infertility. Many variables may influence success rates after intrauterine insemination (IUI), including sperm quality in the native and washed semen sample. Semen analysis has to be performed according to World Health Organization (WHO) criteria.[12] Standard procedures in semen analysis include evaluation of sperm concentration, motility, morphology and vitality. Although the WHO classification suggests accuracy, the relevance for the prognosis of the couple and the choice of treatment is poor.[13]

In a systemic review by Ombelet—The four sperm parameters that were most frequently examined during semen analysis and above which IUI pregnancy outcome is significantly improved were the following: (i) inseminating motile count after washing: cut-off value between 0.8 and 5 million; (ii) sperm morphology using strict criteria: cut-off value $\geq 4\%$

normal morphology; (iii) total motile sperm count in the native sperm sample: cut-off value of 5–10 million; and (iv) total motility in the native sperm sample: threshold value of 30%.

According to Ombelet et al an inseminating motile count (IMC) of 1 million can be used as a reasonable threshold level above which IUI can be performed with acceptable pregnancy rates.[14]

Total motile sperm count (TMSC): TMC gets around the problem of fluctuating ejaculate volumes by combining the ejaculate volume, sperm concentration, motility to provide the total number of motile sperms in the entire ejaculate. If the TMC is 20 million sperm or less, there is likely to be significant male factor infertility. Men with a TMC consistently less than 5 million are said to have severe male factor Infertility.[15]

The value of the postwash TMSC at insemination relies on the enhancement of patient selection by identifying couples that are unlikely to conceive with IUI due to its high specificity. Postwash TMC could be used in counseling patients for the selection of better treatment.[16]

According to the new and updated recommendations published in the NICE clinical guidelines, IUI is not recommended anymore for unexplained and mild male factor infertility (NICE guidelines, 2013). For people with unexplained infertility, mild endometriosis or mild male factor infertility, who are having regular unprotected sexual intercourse, it is advised not to offer IUI routinely, either with or without ovarian stimulation, but advise them to try to conceive for a total of 2 years before IVF will be considered.[6] Despite the NICE recommendations, it can be expected that artificial insemination with husband's semen remains a widely used treatment option for many couples with unexplained infertility, cervical factor subfertility, physiological or psychological sexual dysfunction and mild-to-moderate male subfertility.

When the average TMSC was, 10 million, pregnancy rates were very low after IUI whether or not controlled ovarian hyperstimulation was performed in the woman. Above this threshold, IUI pregnancy rates reached a plateau with no further increases in the pregnancy rate noted at higher values. In addition, when the average TMSC was above 30 million, higher pregnancy rates were noted when controlled ovarian hyperstimulation was used in conjunction with the IUI cycle as compared with natural cycle IUI.[17]

Receptive Endometrium

Endometrial thickness and pattern on the day of the spontaneous LH surge or hCG administration are intimately associated with implantation success or failure. Implantation does not occur, or occurs at a reduced rate per follicle, if the endometrium lacks a triple-line pattern on the day of hCG administration. Abnormal patterns seen at this time include fluid within the endometrial cavity, which if persistent is incompatible with implantation; fluid collection within the fallopian tube and small polyps that were not visible earlier in the cycle. A homogeneous pattern may be an indication of endometrial or uterine pathology.

In a meta-analysis conducted recently stated that there is no association between endometrial thickness and pregnancy rate so it does not seems to be a predictor for success in IUI. Thin endometrium is clinically more relevant in IVF cycles than in IUI.[18]

COUNSELING

People who experience fertility problems should be offered counseling because fertility problems themselves, and the investigation and treatment of fertility problems, can cause psychological stress. The objectives of counseling are to provide emotional support, to alleviate their stress, to impart knowledge about their specific problem, need for the procedure and the procedure itself, and cost of the treatment and likelihood of success.

Counseling should be provided by counselor who is not directly involved in the management of the individual's with fertility problems.

Couples should have the opportunity to make informed decisions regarding their care and treatment.

Types of Counseling

The HFEA Code of Practice (HFEA 2008) identifies three distinct types of counseling:

a. Implication Counseling

To enable couple to understand the implication of the treatment for themselves, their family and for the child born as a result.

b. Support Counseling

To give emotional support and it is to be offered before, during and after investigation and treatment, irrespective of the outcome of these procedures. People who experience fertility problems should be informed that they may find it helpful to contact a fertility support group.

c. Therapeutic Counseling

Therapeutic counseling aims to help people cope with the consequences of infertility and treatment, to resolve problems which these may cause, and to adjust their expectations so that they can cope with the outcome of treatment, whatever that may be.

Counseling Regarding Donor Insemination

For most couples it might be very difficult to accept donor sperm as an option. All possible modalities of treatment and the possible costs should be put forth to them. Couples should also be assured of complete confidentiality, and informed that all sperm donors are now comprehensively screened for genetic and infective conditions. Couples should also be informed how the donor is to be matched to their own characteristics, the cost of treatment, and the probability of success, and physical and psychological implications of treatment, the potential for complications to occur and the likelihood of their occurrence. The sample will be from an anonymous donor and anonymity will be maintained lifelong. It is not obligatory for the couple to disclose to the child that it is born out of donor insemination. The couple should decide it themselves what treatment they want to opt for.

INFORMED CONSENTS

Taking an informed consent is essential step in all procedures. Written, well-informed valid time consent in regional language should be taken from both the partners in the format given by ICMR [supplementary document attached]. The clinic must ensure that patient are well-informed about the treatment being offered to them, the reason of suggesting a particular form of treatment, the advantages or disadvantages, alternate therapies available, the success rates, the time-required, possible complications, postprocedure care and cost. This should be counter-signed by the doctor attending. In case of donor IUI, a separate consent form is required this is to be signed by both partners. If this procedure is done without the consent of husband, it might be a ground for divorce in the court of law.

In view of the fact that IUI is a relatively simple procedure compared with *in vitro* fertilization (IVF), its popularity as a treatment option for certain groups of infertile couples is increasing, since it is intermediate between the simpler ovulation induction (OI) and the more 'high-tech' IVF. This is particularly so important in developing countries, where facilities for IVF may be limited and the cost of treatment by IVF is a major issue.

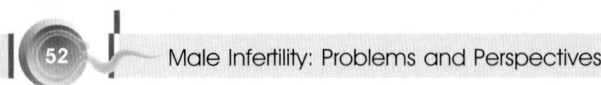

Form E: Consent for Artificial Insemination or Intrauterine Insemination with Husband's Semen/Sperm

We,_____ and _____, being husband and wife and both of legal age, authorize Dr _____ to inseminate the wife artificially or intrauterine with semen or sperm of husband for achieving conception.

We understand that even though the insemination may be repeated as often as recommended by the doctor, there is no guarantee or assurance that pregnancy or a live birth will result.

We have also been told that the outcome of pregnancy may not be the same as those of the general patient population, e.g. in respect of abortion, multiple pregnancies, anomalies or complications of pregnancy or delivery.

The procedure carried out does not ensure a positive result, nor does it guarantee a mentally and physically normal child. This consent holds good for all the cycles performed at the clinic.

Endorsement by the Assisted Reproductive Technology Clinic

I/we have personally explained to_____ and_____ the details and implications of his/her/their signing this consent/approval form, and made sure to the extent humanly possible that he/she/they understand these details and implications.

Signed_____ (Husband) _____ (Wife)

Name and signature of the doctor _____

Name, address and signature
of the witness from the clinic _____

Name and address of the ART clinic _____

Dated: _____

Form F: Consent for Artificial Insemination or Intrauterine Insemination with Donor Semen

We, _____ and _____, being husband and wife and both of legal age, authorize Dr_____ to inseminate the wife artificially or intrauterine with semen or sperm of a donor (ART bank's no._____; obtained from_____ ART bank with valid registration no._____) for achieving conception.

We understand that even though the insemination may be repeated as often as recommended by the doctor, there is no guarantee or assurance that pregnancy or a live birth will result.

We have also been told that the outcome of pregnancy may not be the same as those of the general patient population, e.g. in respect of abortion, multiple pregnancies, anomalies or complications of pregnancy or delivery.

We declare that we shall not attempt to find out the identity of the donor. I, the husband, also declare that should my wife bear any child or children as a result of such insemination(s), such child or children shall be as my own and shall be my legal heir(s).

The procedure carried out does not ensure a positive result, nor does it guarantee a mentally and physically normal child. This consent holds good for all the cycles performed at the clinic.

Endorsement by the Assisted Reproductive Technology Clinic

I/we have personally explained to_____ and_____ the details and implications of his/her/their signing this consent/approval form, and made sure to the extent humanly possible that he/she/they understand these details and implications.

Signed_____ (Husband) _____ (Wife)

Name and signature of the doctor _____

Name, address and signature
of the witness from the clinic _____

Name and address of the ART clinic _____

Dated: _____

REFERENCES

1. Prietal G, Van der ven, Kerbs D. Artificial insemination: noninvasive management of subfertile couples. Manual on Assisted Reproduction, 2nd Edn. Berlin: Springer 2000;601.
2. Cantineau AE, Janssen MJ, Cohlen BJ, Allersma T. Synchronised approach for intrauterine insemination in subfertile couples. Cochrane Database of Systematic Reviews 2014, Issue 12.
3. MME van Rumste, IM Custers, F van der Veen, M van Wely, JLH Evers, BWJ Mol. The influence of the number of follicles on pregnancy rates in intrauterine insemination with ovarian stimulation: a meta-analysis, Human Reproduction Update, 2008;14(6):563–70,
4. Banker M, Patel A, Deshmukh A, et al. Comparison of Effectiveness of Different Protocols Used for Controlled Ovarian Hyperstimulation in Intrauterine Insemination Cycle. J Obstet Gynecol India 2018;68:65. https://doi.org/10.1007/s13224–017–1054-8.
5. Chaudhary K, Suri V, Dhaliwal LK, et al. Comparison of the efficacy of letrozole and low-dose gonadotropin combination with clomiphene and low-dose gonadotropin combination as a controlled ovarian stimulation regime prior to intrauterine insemination in patients with unexplained infertility. Fertil Sci Res. 2014;1:98.
6. National Institute for Health and Care Excellence (NICE). Fertility: assessment and treatment for people with fertility problems. NICE Clinical Guidelines, No. 156 (2004, amended 2013) (updated September 2017). Available at www.nice.org.uk/guidance/cg156
7. Goverde AJ, Lambalk CB, McDonnell J, Schats R, Homburg R, Vermeiden JP. Further considerations on natural or mild hyperstimulation cycles for intrauterine insemination treatment: effects on pregnancy and multiple pregnancy rates, Hum Reprod 2005;20:3141–6.
8. Practice Committee of the American Society for Reproductive Medicine. Role of tubal surgery in the era of assisted reproductive technology: a committee opinion. Fertil Steril. 2015 Jun; 103(6): e37–43.
9. Papaioannou S, Bourdrez P, Varma R, Afnan M, Mol BW, Coomarasamy A. Tubal evaluation in the investigation of subfertility: a structured comparison of tests. BJOG 2004; 111:1313–21.
10. Serene Liqing Lim, Jacqueline Jingjin Jung, Su LingYu, Hemashree. A comparison of hysterosalpingo-foam sonography (HyFoSy) and hysterosalpingo-contrast-sonography with saline medium (HyCoSy) in the assessment of tubal patency. European Journal of Obstetrics and Gynecology and Reproductive Biology 2015;195: 168–70.
11. Rajagopal V, Chamberlain S, Weston G. Intrauterine insemination (IUI) in patients with single patent tube. A retrospective review to analyze cancellation rate, pregnancy rate and to improve pretreatment counseling. Fertility and Sterility 2014;102(3):e219.
12. World Health Organisation: Department of Reproductive Health and Research WHO laboratory manual for the examination and processing of human semen, (5th edn.), 2010.
13. Hamilton JA, Cissen M, Brandes M, Smeenk JM, de Bruin JP, Kremer JA, Nelen WL, Hamilton CJ. Total motile sperm count: a better indicator for the severity of male factor infertility than the WHO sperm classification system. Hum Reprod 2015;30:1110–21.
14. Ombelet W, Dhont N, Thijssen A, Bosmans E, Kruger T. Semen quality and prediction of IUI success in male subfertility: a systematic review. eprod Biomed Online. 2014;28(3):300–9.
15. Miller DC, Hollenbeck BK, Smith GD, Randolph JF, Christman GM, Smith YR, Lebovic DI, Ohl DA. Processed total motile sperm count correlates with pregnancy outcome after intrauterine in semination. Urology 2002;60(3):497–501.
16. Van Weert JM, Repping S, Van Voorhis BJ, van der Veen F, Bossuyt PM, Mol BW. Performance of the postwash total motile sperm count as a predictor of pregnancy at the time of intrauterine insemination: a meta-analysis. Fertil Steril 2004;82:612–20.
17. Mehrannia T. The relationship between total motile sperm count and pregnancy rate after intrauterine insemination. Pak J Med Sci 2006; 22(3):223–7.
18. Weiss NS, van Vliet MN, Limpens J, Hompes PGA, Lambalk CB , Mochtar MH, van der Veen F , Mol BWJ, van Wely M; Endometrial thickness in women undergoing IUI with ovarian stimulation. How thick is too thin? A systematic review and meta-analysis, Human Reproduction, 2017;32(5)1009–18.

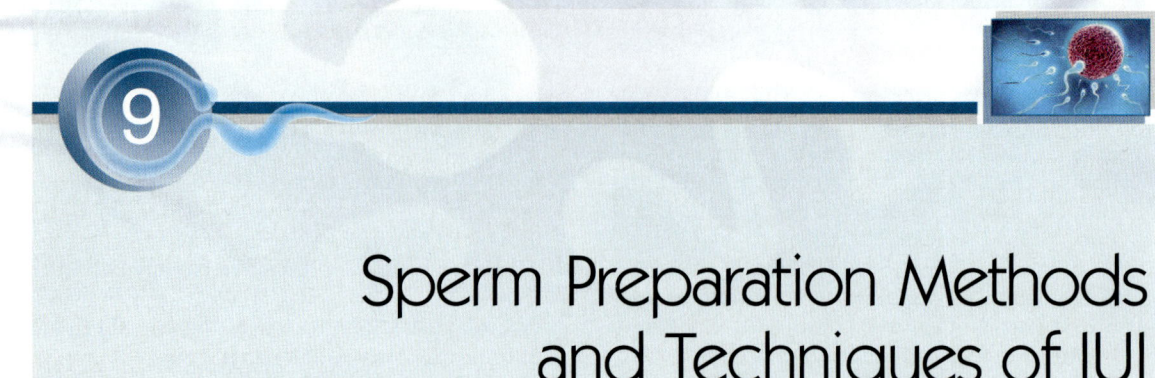

Sperm Preparation Methods and Techniques of IUI

Surykant Hayatnagarkar

Intrauterine insemination (IUI) as a therapy for infertility was introduced mainstream in early 70s in Europe and USA and early 80s in India.[1] Despite ups and downs of hopes, of an all-round therapy for infertility, subsequent advent of *in vitro* fertilization and intracytoplasmic insemination, it has remained primary line therapy for majority of couples seeking treatment for infertility. Intrauterine insemination became a popular therapy after advent of improved methods of semen processing.

The treatment of infertility is mostly empirical and intrauterine insemination or IUI is the most important tool available for active intervention in the treatment of infertile couples. It is technically simple, easy to carry out in a simple clinical set-up, yet the most cost effective treatment compared to other high cost therapies like IVF, ICSI, etc.

Recent advances in fertility research and development of improved techniques for processing and preservation of sperms has improved the success rates in artificial insemination. Sperm processing is the cornerstone of all artificial reproductive techniques and more so for intrauterine insemination. Sperm processing methods basically must emulate the transport mechanism of sperms in female genital tract.

Sperm Transport in Female Genital Tract

Mature sperm ejaculated in vagina are suspended in accessory gland secretions which protect against hostile acidic vaginal environment. Cervical mucus also is hostile throughout the cycle except at the time of ovulation, when it becomes thick, sticky and copious. It dips into the fornix also. Motile sperm quickly penetrate cervical mucus around the time of ovulation, escaping from vaginal acidic atmosphere. Only periovulatory cervical mucus is receptive to sperm. Cervical mucus also works as sperm reservoir. From there they are slowly released to uterus and finally swim to fallopian tubes. Out of 100–500 million sperms ejaculated in vagina few thousands only can reach the fallopian tubes.[2] Thus cervical mucus acts as a filter allowing only normal motile sperms to enter uterus and filtering out nonmotile, nonfunctional sperm, contaminating cells, debris and seminal plasma.

Freshly ejaculated sperm are incapable of fertilization and undergo series of structural and chemical changes, during passage through cervical mucus, termed capacitation. This is characterized by hyperactivation motility.[3]

While doing intrauterine insemination this cervical mucus function is bypassed by depositing sperm directly into uterus. So any sperm processing method has to emulate the actions of cervical mucus to be effective.

Rationale for Doing IUI

The inability of sperm to successfully reach the site of fertilization may be due to various female as well as male factors. Oligospermia, asthenospermia, teratozoospermia, inability to penetrate cervical mucus are some of the important male factors. Female factors include hostile cervical mucus and anatomical defects in the female genital tract. These factors will decrease availability of sperm at the site of fertilization and by semen processing and intrauterine insemination availability of sperm in fallopian tubes can be increased resulting in optimization of fertilization.

Rationale for IUI
• Optimization of gamete availability at the site of fertilization • Reduction in distance traveled by sperm • Tackling of occult seminal problems • Optimization of ovulation and endometrium.

Rationale for Sperm Processing

In order to perform intrauterine insemination, it is necessary to separate motile spermatozoa from unwanted fractions like, seminal plasma, debris, nonmotile and dead sperms and leucocytes. All the effects of cervical mucus must be imitated to get effective processing. At the same time, majority of the motile sperms present in available sample for processing should reach the final processed volume so as to get maximum number of normal sperms ready to compete for fertilization. The processing should induce gentle capacitation so that sperms which are directly transferred to uterus, should be ready with fertilizing ability.[4]

Ideal goals for sperm processing
• Select highest number of motile sperms • Remove seminal plasma and prostaglandins • Remove dead, damaged and abnormal sperms • Remove white cells and round cells • Induce capacitation and hyperactivation.

Sperm Processing Methods[4]

Sperm processing methods have evolved from very simple wash-centrifugation procedures[5] to complex density gradients[6, 7] and specia-

lized devices based on various techniques. Broadly now most of the processing techniques are based on principles like innate motility of sperm or density differences in normal and dead sperms. Majority of the specialized 'KITS' are based on simple techniques but use complex methods and devices to make them unique. They do not provide any specific advantage over the technique they are based on.

Sperm processing methods

• Simple washing
  – Wash and spin
    Methods using sperm motility
    Swim-up from neat semen (layering)
    Swim up from pellet
    Self-migration and sedimentation
    Swim-up from ejaculate into hyaluronic acid column
• Methods based on density differences
  – Percoll, pure sperm, Silane coated silica gel
  – Polysaccharide or isolate gradients
  – Ficoll gradient
  – Nycodenz
• Methods depending on other physical characteristics
  – Glass wool filtration
  – Glass bead separation
  – Sephadex columns.

Simple Centrifugation Wash Method

This simplest processing method first introduced by Hanson and Rock in 1951.[8] Technique is especially useful in very simple set-up. Procedure involves 2–3 times dilution of liquified semen with nutrient medium, followed by centrifugation at approximately 300 g for 10 minutes. Supernatant is removed; and pellet is resuspended in fresh nutrient medium. This is again centrifuged to wash out remaining seminal plasma and finally resuspended in 0.5 ml of fresh medium. This fraction is used for insemination.

The main disadvantage of this simplistic wash procedure is that not only normal sperm but all the debris, nonmotile sperm and leucocytes are tightly packed in the pellet and

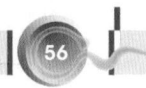

all this contamination forms part of inseminate. This contaminating debris is potentially dangerous due to formation of reactive oxygen species which can irreversibly damage sperm membrane leading to failure of fertilization.[9, 10]

This method can be used for samples with minimal quantity of debris and normal motile sperms, albeit low counts.

Swim-up Methods

Due to potential problems inherent to the simple wash and spin method, the methods using sperm innate motility characteristics became quickly popular. Sperm migration methods are based on same property of sperm by which it penetrates and migrates through the cervical mucus, and debris, nonmotile sperm, other cellular components are left behind.

Drevius (1971)[5] first time demonstrated sperm can be separated by swim-up method from mixed population pellet due to ability of sperm to migrate from one medium to another, due to natural forward progressive motile nature of normal sperm. Based on this premise Lopata et al (1976),[11] used swim method for patient treatment.

This class of migration methods involve either swim-up or swim down of motile sperm directly from semen, or from washed pellet of sperm to fresh nutrient medium.

Swim up directly from semen is simplest way to harvest good population of motile sperm, and it is rapid effective method to obtain good yield from normal samples.[12]

The semen is divided into different tubes 0.5 ml each and number of tubes can be setup depending on amount of semen available. The semen is layered over with nutrient medium equal quantity and the tubes are capped and kept in incubator for 45 to 90 minutes at 37°C. The tubes can be kept in inclined position to increase the surface area available for sperm to migrate.

After incubation supernatant containing motile sperm migrated from seminal plasma is harvested and pooled into a conical bottom centrifuge tube. Tube is centrifuged for 10 minutes at 300 g and pellet containing highly motile sperm is resuspended in 0.5 ml fresh nutrient medium and examined to calculate yield.

Another method involves initial wash and centrifugation and use of pellet to layer nutrient medium.[11] The tube with undisturbed pellet and layered nutrient medium is incubated for up to one hour. Supernatant containing motile sperm is then separated to another tube and centrifuged for 10 minutes at 300 g. This pellet is finally resuspended in 0.5 ml fresh nutrient medium and examined. This procedure of swim-up from washed pellet is good for semen samples with normal or high sperm concentration, normal motility and clean cell free semen.

Samples with high debris and other cellular components can induce formation of free oxygen radicals if packed into pellet along with normal sperm.

In terms of efficiency of motile sperm recovery, swim-up methods rely most on quality (speed) of motility, the quantity of motile sperm in the original sample and the skill of the technician in the procedure. It is preferred technique with sample relatively free of contaminating cells and debris and with high sperm concentration. (Centola, 2005).[13]

Yield of swim-up being low, procedure can be used in good samples only when IUI is considered.

Density Gradient Centrifugation

The density gradient procedure is the most popular method used to prepare semen for insemination.[14] Percoll, a product of PVP coated silica particles, was the most widely used density gradient solution in early 1990s until it was declared not for human use. Subsequently silane coated silica particles gradients were developed.

Density gradient separation of sperm is based on sperm size, motility and density.

(Ruiz et al. 2003) The gradient media used should have minimal or no osmotic effect, low viscosity and high specific gravity.

The method is also called discontinuous gradient separation as two different concentrations of gradient typically 90% and 45% are used by gently layering one on top of other thus producing distance density layers (discontinuous). The specimen is layered on top of the gradient and centrifuged at 300–500 g for 20 minutes. Centrifugal force propels cellular components including debris, motile and nonmotile sperm and other cellular components downwards in contact with density gradient medium. Motile sperm can pass through easily due to higher dense nature and other components lag behind or held in upper layers or fluid interface. Only good normal dense motile sperms finally reach the pellet and other components are held up at various heights. Exposure to 'multiple' layers of density gradient effective 'cleans' the semen sample and concentrates highly motile sperm fraction at the bottom of the tube.[15]

The supernatant including interfaces is removed gently using pipette and the pellet then washed in fresh nutrient medium and centrifuged for 5–10 minutes to get clean pellet. The final pellet is then suspended in 05 ml fresh nutrient medium.

Recently a single gradient layer has been used for sperm preparation. Single interface is used for routine processing of samples. Double or multiple layer gradients are used for samples with low count, low motility and high debris (Gliedt et al. 2003).[15]

However, a single gradient is enough for processing almost all specimen for routine IUI, it is most cost-effective and results in recovery of adequate numbers of motile sperm.[16]

High semen viscosity is also an important problem in semen processing. Many a times it become difficult to process sample using swip-up technique and various methods like immediate dilution with nutrient medium, chymotrypsin treatment, passing through 20 gauge needle repeatedly all have been tried with variable results.

Density gradient centrifugation can be used for such samples without much difficulty without fear of any sperm damage easily.

Processing of Cryopreserved Samples

Donor insemination using frozen samples is very common technique. Presently most of the samples available are pre-processed and cryopreserved using IUI ready cryoprotectant. But in initial period samples were frozen with seminal plasma and needed to be processed before IUI.

Spermatozoa which are cryopreserved are variously damaged by the freezing and thawing process. It is therefore necessary not to manipulate too much while processing. Simple wash and spin can be used to process these samples if post thaw motility is good, otherwise it is best to process such samples using density gradient as density gradients provide good cushioning to sperms subjected to centrifugation.

Processing of Retrograde Ejaculates

Retrograde ejaculation occurs when semen is forced back into urinary bladder rather than regular ejaculation out of urethra at the time of orgasm. This can happen in various conditions including diabetes, some medicines or spinal injuries. As the semen enters bladder, normal acidic urine makes them immotile or dead. So there is need to handle these patients in specialized way.[17]

Sperm can be recovered immediately following retrograde ejaculation and used for IUI or other ART procedures, provided urine is alkalinized for at least 4 hours prior to the ejaculation and small quantity of urine is collected immediately after orgasm. Bladder is voiced immediately after ejaculation and is immediately diluted using nutrient medium. It is centrifuged using as many tubes required at 300 g for 10 minutes and pellets are resuspended and pooled using small amount of fresh medium. After examination it can be further concentrated to 0.5 ml fresh medium and used for insemination. It it contains large amount of debris and contaminating cells density gradient using mini gradient with give clean motile sperm for insemination.

Sperm Processing Media[12,13]

Drevious (1971) demonstrated movement of sperms in nutrient media and potential of using motile only fraction of sperm for examination and insemination. This opened up the field for development of various sperm processing techniques. All require some nutrient media which should be of physiological pH, osmolarity and composition of natural body fluids at the same time supporting and nurturing the sperm function.

Initially simple Ringer's lactate was used and found to give good separation. Later on specific tissue culture media like HAM F10, EBSS, DMEM, Tyrode's buffer, BWW medium were all variously introduced. All are now replaced by defined simple media based on Quinn's formulation which now is termed Human Tubal Fluid Medium. This medium is based on tests done on follicular fluid and also contains buffers like bicarbonate requiring CO_2 for stabilization of pH or HEPES buffer which does not require CO_2 for stabilization. Use of HEPES became common for IUI as it requires simple incubator and there is no specific need for CO_2 incubation as in IVF and ET procedures. The media need protein supplements and most physiological supplement is human albumin or synthetic serum substitutes. It is essential for sperm survival and initiation of capacitation. Most commonly albumin is added in proportion of 3–5 mg/ml of medium. Antitbiotics like gentamicin can be added to reduce chances of infection due to contamination from semen sample.

Initially all the media were prepared in house from either dry powder mix or using individual components. It required stringent production of pyrogen free water, equipment to adjust pH, osmolarity and quality testing.

Quickly, the home made reagents were replaced by commercially produced stringent quality controlled reagents and media. Many different commercial brands are now available in market to choose from. Most essential quality criteria for choosing media are proper pH indicated by phenol red indicator in the medium, osmolarity and should be endotoxin free. Smaller single use unit packing will be preferable over larger multidose units due to chances of contamination during removal for each processing. All the media are stored in refrigerator until use. Prior to use all the media required for use must be brought to 37°C in incubator or heating block.

For density gradient separation initially percoll was the choice gradient. Percoll or its substitutes are available in form of specific density silica gel particles coated with PVP or silane and are less than 25 mOsm. To make initial isotonic medium one has to use 10X medium and 100 ml 10X medium is mixed with 900 ml density gradient to make isotonic stock. This is further diluted to required strengths using regular medium. Generally used percentages are 90%, 60%, 45%, etc.

Equipment Requirements and How to Set up IUI Lab[13]

Setting up of IUI program in any clinical set-up is rather a simple job now as the equipment required is available a plenty, and very cost-effective too. Good centrifuge having RPM meter, timer and swingout rotor is essential for all the processing methods. Centrifugation speed to g force calculation varies from machine to machine and while setting up the processing lab it is necessary to set proper RPM to get proper g force. It can be calculated from the manufacturer's manual. Lowest possible g force or RPM to achieve desired separation should be used to reduce chances of damage to sperm during centrifugation. For semen analysis before processing and checking after processing a good compound microscope is essential. Phase contrast attachment is desirable as it gives good visualization of sperms in physiological state. Its good to have a trinocular head and digital camera in the third port for visualizing on screen or laptop as well as to create visual record of the sperm motility and other examinations.

Simple incubator, dry bath incubator, test tube warmer block are good for warming nutrient media and samples at 37°C. Swim up and storage of prepared samples can be done in same equipment.

Sterile supplies are essential to perform all the necessary processes including test tubes, pipettes, droppers, syringes, catheters, etc.

The IUI lab should be specifically designed to take into consideration all the requirements, processing methods to be used and the work load. Lab should be equipped with general furnishing like small wall cupboard, refrigerator, tables with solid base scratch free surface preferable with 6–8" working length. Laminar air flow bench is also essential to create dust free atmosphere to work with opened media and samples including all the manipulations. Microscope and centrifuge must be placed on different table or work benches as centrifuges can create vibrations which will impede the visualization in the microscope.

Equipment and supplies for IUI lab

- Trinocular microscope with digital camera
- Incubator or dry bath test tube warmer set at 37°C
- Sperm counting chamber
- Centrifuge with RPM meter, timer and swing out rotor
- Refrigerator
- Laminar flow bench
- Test tube racks
- Sterile pipettes, test tubes, sample collection containers
- IUI canula
- Gloves, spirit, sterilium, swabs, etc.

CONCLUSIONS

It is relatively easy to set-up a sperm preparation laboratory and perform sperm preparation for IUI.

It is difficult to identify a technique that should be used for all types of specimen, but it is necessary to determine method of choice individually tailored to the quality of specimen. It depends not only on sperm concentration, motility, morphology and semen volume but also on results of previous analyses, processing results and quality of sample available for processing at present time.

No single processing method is superior and technique that yields most normal motile sperm needs to be used.

It is very easy to master various techniques easily but many a times deviant samples showing severe oligospermia, asthenospermia, high viscosity can pose challenge to average technician and such specimen need to be referred to specialized andrology laboratories dealing with IVF. Success of IUI programs not only depend on mastering sperm preparation techniques but also on decision-making on preparation of the couple for IUI.

REFERENCES

1. Ombelet W, Van Robays J. Artificial Insemination History: Hurdles and milestones. Facts Views Vis Obgyn 2015;7:137–43.
2. Settlage DSF, Motoshima M. Tredway DR. Sperm Transport from the external os to the fallopian tubes in women: a time and quantitation study. Fertil Steril 1973;24:655–61.
3. Kupker W, Diedrich K, Edwards RG. Ptinciples of mammalian fertilization. Hum Reprod 1998;13:20–32.
4. Byrd W. Processing human semen for insemination comparison of methods. In: Centola GM, Ginsburg KA, eds. Evaluation and treatment of the Infertile Male. Cambrodge: Cambridge University Press, 1996:6–18.
5. Drevius LO. The Sperm-Rise test, J. Reprod. Fert 1971;24:427–9.
6. Morshedi M, Duran HE, Taylor S, Oehninger S. Efficasy and pregnancy outcome of two methods of spem preparation for intrauterine insemination: a prospective randomized study. Fertil Steril 2003;79:1625–32.

7. Sharma RK, Seifarth K, Garlak D, Agarwal A. Conparison of three sperm separation media. Int J Fertil Women's Med 1999;44:163–7.

8. Hanson FM, Rock J. Artificial insemination with husband's sperm. Fertil Steril 1951;2:162–74.

9. Aitken RJ, Gordon E, Harkiss D, et al. Relative impact of oxidative stress on function competence and genomic integrity of human spermatozoa. Biol Reprof 1998;59:1037–46.

10. Shekarriz M, DeWire DM, Thomas AJ, Agarwal A. A method of human semen centrifugation to minimize the iatrogenic sperm injuries caused by reactive oxygen species. Eur Urol 1995;28: 31–5.

11. Lopata A, Patullo MJ, Chang A, James B. A method for collecting motile spermatozoa from human semen. Fertil Steril 1976;27:677–84.

12. Mortimer D, Mortimer ST. Methods of sperm preparation for assisted reproduction. Ann Acad Med Sing 1992;21:517–24.

13. Centola GM. Sperm preparation for insemination. In: Patton PF, BattagliaDF, ed. Office Andrology. Totowa NJ: Humana Press 2005;39–52.

14. Ruiz A, Jayendran RS. Sperm processing procedure for intrauterine insemination. In: Jayendran RS (Ed). Sperm collection and processing methods. Cambridge: Cambridge University Press 2003;123–40.

15. Gliedt D, Reed MI. Preparation of gametes for assisted reproductive technologies. In: Andrology and Embryology Review Course Material. Chicago IL; American Association of Bioanalysts, 2003;8.1–8.58.

16. Centola GM, Herko R, Andolina E, Weisensel S. Comparison of sperm separation methods: Effect on recovery, motility, motion parameters and hyperactivation. Fertil Steril 1998;70:1173–5.

17. Olmstead SS, Dubin NH, Cone RA, Moench TR. The rate at which human sperm are immobilized and killed by mild acidity. Fertil Steril 2000; 73:687–93.

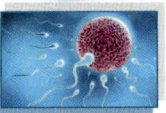

Factors Influencing Success of IUI

Hrishikesh D Pai, Manisha Kundnani, Nandita Palshetkar, Rishma Dhillon Pai and Rohan Palshetkar

Intrauterine insemination (IUI) is often the first line of treatment offered to many infertile couples. The procedure offers many advantages of being simple, easy, relatively economical, and less invasive and needs minimal infrastructure. It also has a good compliance rates and there are few dropouts. The success rates however vary and there are many factors which can influence the success of this treatment. Various studies have reported pregnancy rates per cycle between 8 and 22%.[1] It has been seen that most couples who get pregnant do so within first 4 cycles and the success rates usually plateaus after these many attempts.

There are many factors which can influence the success rate of IUI treatment. The can be broadly categorized as the patient related factors or the procedure related factors.

Patient related factors are:
- Age of the female and the male partner
- Cause of infertility
- Duration of infertility
- Semen parameters.

Procedure related factors are:
- Controlled ovarian stimulation
- Number of preovulatory follicles
- Days of abstinence
- Sperm processing methods
- Sperm preparation time
- Number of inseminations
- Insemination technique

- Number of inseminations per cycle
- Type of catheter
- Post IUI rest
- Luteal phase support.

Patient Related Factors

Age of the Female Partner

Age of the women is the single most important factor influencing success rate after any infertility treatment. Younger women have better success rates compared to elder women and a significant fall in success rate is observed after the age of 35. In a study conducted by Schorsch et al 4246 insemination cycles were analyzed and it was observed that the best pregnancy rates with IUI are achieved in women less than 25 years of age and patients age had a statistically measurable impact on the pregnancy rates.[2] Another study conducted by Merviel et al reported best success rates in women less than 30 years of age.[3]

Age of the Male Partner

Decreased androgen levels and deterioration of semen quality has been observed in males of advanced age. Advanced paternal age (APA) is also known to influence the DNA integrity of sperms, increase in telomere length and is known to have epigenetic effects.[4] These changes can lead to reduced fertility, increase the incidence of pregnancy complications and can also have adverse effect on the offspring. Dunson et al observed that

Table 10.1: Effect of etiology on success rate with IUI	
Infertility etiology	Pregnancy rate
Unexplained	22.6%
Mild male factor	18.8%
Anovulation	12.4%
Endometriosis	6.5%
Tubal factor	7.6%
Combined factors	9.7%

after controlling for the female age, the time to achieve pregnancy and the rate of conception were adversely affected by the advanced paternal age.[5]

Cause of Infertility

The cause of infertility has been observed to influence the success rates of IUI significantly. Those with cervical factor, unexplained infertility, anovulation and sexual dysfunction have better success rates.[6] Mentanaro et al in a step wise regression analysis observed that a female diagnosis of endometriosis and tubal factor has a negative impact on the probability of pregnancy after IUI (risk ratio 0.18) compared to other factors.[7]

Duration of Infertility

Impact of duration of infertility on pregnancy rates has been studied by many researchers, the results are however conflicting. Ashrafi et al, Hansen et al, Kamath et al observed that prolonged duration of infertility is associated with decreased success rates after IUI.[8–10] Zainul et al and Tay et al however did not find any significant difference in pregnancy rates associated with duration of infertility.[11,12]

Semen Parameters

Semen parameters like count, motility and morphology are important determinants of success after IUI. The sperm factors most frequently correlated with success rates are sperm morphology by the strict criteria, total motile sperm count, inseminating motile count, and the total motility. Van Waart and

Ombelet et al observed that more than 4% normal morphology using the strict criteria is needed for optimal IUI results.[13, 14] Another study conducted by Shibahara et al observed the pregnancy rate per IUI cycle of 3.8%, 18.5%, 29.9% in patients with sperm morphology with <4%, 4–9%, >9% normal forms respectively.[15]

The other important sperm parameter significantly influencing the success rate is the total motile sperm count and the inseminating motile count (IMC) (postwash). Ombelet et al suggested a cut off value IMC, TMSC and total motility of 1 million, 5–10 million and 30% respectively for performing IUI with acceptable pregnancy rates.[16]

Couples with teratospermia, with <4% normal sperms or inseminate motile count of less than 1 million, should be considered for ICSI.

Treatment Related Factors

Controlled Ovarian Stimulation

A number of studies have shown that superovulation and IUI gives better results compared to natural cycle IUI. Success rates also vary with the type of stimulation, with gonadotropin stimulated cycles giving better success rates compared to oral ovulogens (clomiphene citrate and letrozole). The combination of gonadotropins and clomiphene/letrozole decreases the dose of gonadotropins needed and gives almost similar pregnancy rates, thereby making it more cost-effective.

Superovulation, however, increases the risk of multiple pregnancies and thus ovarian stimulation should be mild. Ultrasound monitoring is mandatory for every stimulated cycle. A risk analysis conducted by van Rumste et al showed that the aim should be for a maximum of two dominant follicles in order to avoid multiple gestations.[17] An optimal ovarian stimulation should aim at 1 or 2 mature follicles with trilaminar endometrium 7 mm thick,[3] on the day of the trigger .

Alternative measures like cycle cancellation or escape IVF should be adopted if there are 4 or more follicles[3] 14 mm or 8 or more follicles >12 mm on the day of HCG in order to prevent higher order pregnancies.

The addition of GnRh analogs (agonists and antagonists) for IUI stimulation has not shown to improve pregnancy rates and is not cost-effective for all IUI cycles.[18,19] GnRh antagonists can however be added in selected cases with history of premature l h surge and follicular rupture or to avoid IUI on weekends.

Number of Preovulatory Follicles

Pregnancy rates increase with the increase in number of preovulatory cycles. This also lead to increase rates of higher order gestations. Huttenen et al observed maximum pregnancy rates (16.3%, p value = 0.013) with 3 preovulatory follicles on the day of trigger. No improved pregnancy rates were seen after 4 follicles, instead there was a 10 fold increase in multiple pregnancy rates.[20]

Days of Abstinence

A short period of ejaculatory abstinence has been associated with higher pregnancy rates. Marshburn et al and Sukprasert et al in independent studies observed that an ejaculatory abstinence of 2–3 days gives the highest pregnancy rates than longer intervals of abstinence.[21,22]

Sperm Processing Methods

Different methods are used for sperm preparation before IUI including simple wash, swim-up and single and double density centrifugation. Though density gradient centrifugation has been observed to be superior to swim-up and simple wash techniques in obtaining morphologically normal spermatozoa with grade A motility and normal DNA integrity, no significant difference has been observed in the clinical pregnancy rates with different methods of semen preparation.[23] Quality control and quality management are however mandatory in semen preparation with any technique being used.

Sperm Preparation Time

IUI pregnancy rates are enhanced by shorter intervals from semen collection to procedure. Best results are obtained with IUI performed within 90 minutes of collection.[24] Semen specimens should be processed immediately after liquefaction and within 30 minutes of collection and IUI should be performed soon after processing. Longer intervals can have deteriorating effects on semen quality because of fluctuation in temperature and pH or because of contamination.

Timing of Insemination

As oocyte and spermatozoa have limited lifespan, proper timing of IUI is important to achieve pregnancy. IUI can be timed according to LH surge detection or HCG injection. It is mostly scheduled after 36 hours of HCG injection. However, a number of studies have shown that a wider time frame for IUI, from 12–36 hours after HCG injection, does not significantly affect the success rates.[25,26]

Number of Inseminations

A single well-timed insemination is usually recommended. According to the cochrane metanalysis, performing double insemination does not increase the success rates compared to single insemination.[25] A study conducted by Liu et al showed a positive impact of double insemination in couples suffering from male factor infertility.[27] Double IUI as a routine, may increases the cost of treatment and psychological burden on the patient.

IUI under USG Guidance

IUI performed under USG guidance has been observed to not significantly enhance the pregnancy rates.[28,29] USG guidance can sometimes ease the procedure in cases of difficult inseminations.

Type of Catheter

The type of catheter does not seem to have any significant effect on the success rates of IUI.[30] Most clinicians prefer using a semisoft catheter as the procedure is difficult with soft catheter and patient discomfort is higher with hard catheter. Gentle atraumatic technique is the essence of successful IUI.

Post IUI Rest

Saleh et al and Custers et al observed that 10–15 minutes of immobilization after insemination has significant effect on the ongoing pregnancy rates and live birth rates.[31,32]

Luteal Phase Support

A good luteal phase support is necessary for the survival of the early pregnancy and has shown to positively affects the success of COH and IUI cycles. Ovulation induction with multifollicular development is known to alter the endocrine environment and thus has a negative impact on the luteal phase.[33] Seckin et al in a prospective randomized study observed that luteal phase support after intrauterine insemination significantly increased the clinical pregnancy rates (28.2% vs 11.4%, p=0.04) in patients with multifollicular response (>1 dominant follicle).[34]

Other metanalysis conducted by Hill et al and Miralpiex et al also observed significantly higher pregnancy rates in women who received progesterone in the luteal phase compared to those with no luteal phase support.[35,36]

The commonly used drugs for luteal phase support are intravaginal micronized progesterone, oral dydrogestrone or intramuscular progesterone. Recent studies have proved that oral dydrogestrone is as effective as vaginal progesterone for luteal phase support after intrauterine insemination.[37,38]

CONCLUSION

Intrauterine insemination is a valuable first line of treatment of many infertile couples. The current available evidence suggests that success rates are improved with ovulation induction and with IMC above 1 million, morphology score of >4% and total motile sperm count of more than 5 million. The ovarian stimulation should be mild with the aim of achieving maximum of two dominant follicles. A single well-timed IUI is recommended in majority of the couples, except mild male factor where , double IUI may be beneficial. 10–15 minutes of bedrest post-insemination and progesterone supplementation in the luteal phase enhances the success rates.

REFERENCES

1. Cohlen BJ, te Velde ER, van Kooji RJ, et al. Controlled ovarian stimulation and intrauterine insemination for treating male subfertility: a controlled study. Hum Reprod 1998;13:1553–8.
2. Schorcsh M, Homez R, Hann T, Hoelscher-Obermaier J, Seufert R, Skala C. Success rates of inseminations are dependent on maternal age? An analysis of 4246 insemination cycles. Geburtshilfe Frauenheilkd 2013;73(8):808–11.
3. Merviel P, Heraud MH, Grenier N, Lourdel E, Sanquinet P, Copin H. Predictive factors for pregnancy after intrauterine insemination (IUI): an analysis of 1038 cycles and a review of literature. Fertil Steril 2010;93(1):79–88.
4. Sartorius GA, Nieschlag E. paternal age and reproduction, Hum Reprod 2010;16(1):65–79.
5. Dunson DB, Baird DD, Colombo B. Increased infertility with age in men and women. Obstet Gynecol 2004;103:51–6.
6. Khalil MR, Rasmussen PE, Erb K, et al. Homologous IUI. An evaluation of prognostic factors based on review of 2473 cycles. Hum Reprod 1999;14:698–703.
7. Mentanaro GM, Kruger TF, Coetze K, et al. Stepwise regression analysis study to study the male and female factors impacting on pregnancy rates in an IUI programme. Andrologia 2001; 33:135–41.
8. Ashrafi M, Rashidi M, Ghasemi A, et al. The role of infertility etiology in success rate of intrauterine insemination cycles: an evaluation of predictive factors for pregnancy rate, International Journal of Fertility and Sterility, 2013;7(2):100–7.

9. Hansen KR, He AL, Styer AK, et al. Predictors of pregnancy and live-birth in couples with unexplained infertility after ovarian stimulation intrauterine insemination, Fertility and Sterility, 2016;105(6):1575–83.

10. Kamath MS, Bhave PTK, Aleyamma TK, et al. Predictive factors for pregnancy after intrauterine insemination: a prospective study of factors affecting outcome, Journal of Human Reproductive Sciences 2010;3(3):129–34.

11. Zainul MRR, Ong FB, Omar MH, et al. Predictors of intrauterine insemination success, Medical Journal of Malaysia, 2006;61(5):599–607.

12. Tay PY, Raj VR, Kulenthran A, Sitizawiah O. Prognostic factors influencing pregnancy rate after stimulated intrauterine insemination. Medical Journal of Malaysia. 2007;62(4):286–9.

13. Van Waart J, Kruger TF, Lombard CJ, Ombelet W. Predictive value of normal sperm morphology in intrauterine insemination (IUI): a structured literature review. Hum Reprod 2001; 7:495–500.

14. Ombelet W, Deblaere K, Bosmans E, Cox A, Jacobs P, Janssen M, et al. Semen quality and intrauterine insemination. Reprod Biomed Online 2003;7:485–92.

15. Shibahara H, Obara H, Ayustawati, et al. Prediction of pregnancy by IUI using CASA estimates and strict criteria in patients with male factor infertility. Int J Androl 2004;27:63–8.

16. Ombelet W, Vandeput H, Van De Putte G, Cox A, Janssen M, Jacobs P, et al. Intrauterine insemination after ovarian stimulation with clomiphene citrate: predictive potential of inseminating motile count and sperm morphology. Hum Reprod 1997;12:1458–63.

17. van Rumste MM, Custers IM, Van der Veen F, Van Wely M, Evers JL, Mol BW. The influence of the number of follicles on pregnancy rates of intrauterine insemination with ovarian stimulation: a metanaalysis. Hum Reprod Update 2008;14:563-70.

18. Cantineau AE, Cohen BJ, Heineman MJ. Ovarian stimulation protocols (anti-oestrogens, gonadotropins with and without GnRh agonists/antagonists) for intrauterine insemination (IUI) in women with subfertility. Cochrane Database Syst Rev 2007;CD005356.

19. Cantineau AE, Cohen BJ, Klip H, Heineman MJ. The addition of GnRh anatagonists in intrauterine insemination cycles with mild ovarian hyperstimulation does not increase live birth rates-a randomized, double blinded, placebo controlled trial. Hum Reprod 2011;26:1104–11.

20. Huttunen SN, Tomas C, Bloigu R, et al. IUI treatment in subfertility. An analysis of factors affecting outcome. Hum Reprod 1999;14:698–703.

21. Sukprasert M, Wongkularb A, Rattanasiri S, Choktanasiri W, Satirapod C. The Effects of Short Abstinence Time on Sperm Motility, Morphology and DNA mDamage. Andrology 2013;2:1.

22. Marshburn PB, Alanis M, Matthews ML, Usadi R, Papadakis MH, Kullstam S, Hurst BS. A short period of ejaculatory abstinence before intrauterine insemination is associated with higher pregnancy rates. Fertil Steril 2010;93(1):286–8.

23. Boomsma CM, Heineman MJ, Cohlen BJ, Farquhar C, Semen preparation techniques for intrauterine insemination. Cochrane Database Syst Rev 2012.

24. Fauque P, Lehert P, Lamotte M, Bettahar-Lebugle K, Bailly A, Diligent C, Cledat M, Pierrot P, Guenedal M, Sagot P. Clinical success of intrauterine insemination cycles is affected by the sperm preparation time. Fertil Steril 2014;101(6): 1618–23.

25. Cantineau AEP, Heineman MJ, Cohlen BJ. Single versus double intrauterine insemination in stimulated cycles for subfertile couples. Cochrane Database Syst Rev 2009.

26. Haller L, Severac F, Rongieres C, Ohl J, Bettahar K, Lichtblau I, Pirrello O. intra uterine insemination at either 24 or 48 hours after ovulation induction: pregnancy and birth rates. Gynecol Obstet Fertil Senol 2017;45(4):210–4.

27. Liu W, Gong F, Luo K, Lu G. comparing the pregnancy rates of one versus two intrauterine inseminations in male factor and idiopathic infertility. J assist Reprod Genet 2006;23:75–9.

28. Ramon O, Matorras R, Corcostegui B, Meabe A, Burgos J, ExpositoA, Crisol L. Ultrasound guided intrauterine insemination-a randomized controlled trial. Hum Reprod 2009;24:1080.

29. Polat I, Ekiz A, Yildirim G, Sahin O, Ulker V, Alkis I, Tekirdag AI. Ultrasound guided intrauterine insemination versus blind intrauterine insemination: a randomized controlled trial. Clin Exp Obstet Gynecol 2015;42(5):657–62.

30. Ahmed MA, Ragana TM, Hesham GA, et al. IUI catheters for assisted reproduction: a systematic review and metaanalysis. Hum Reprod 2006;21: 1961–7.

31. Saleh A, Tan SL, Biljan MM, Tulandi T. A randomized study of the effect of 10 minutes of

bed rest after intrauterine insemination. Fertil Steril 2000;74:509–11.

32. Custers IM, Flierman PA, Maas P, Cox T, Van Dessel TJ, Gerards MH, et al. Immobilisation versus immediate mobilization after intrauterine insemination: randomized control trial. BMJ 2009; 339:b4080.

33. Lo Monte G, Piva I, Bazzan E, Marci R, Ogrin C. Luteal phase support for assisted reproductive technologies: between past, present and future. Minerva Endocrinol 2013;38:401–14.

34. Seckin B, Turkcapar F, Yildiz Y, Senturk B, Yilmaz N, Gulerman C. Effect of luteal phase support with vaginal progesteronein intrauterine insemi-nation cycles with regard to follicular response: a prospective randomized trial. J Reprod Med 2014;59:260–6.

35. Hill MJ, Whitcomb BW, Lewis TD, WuM, Terry N, DeCherney AH, et al. Progesterone luteal support after ovulation induction and intra-uterine insemination: a systematic review and meta-analysis. Fertil Steril 2013;100:1373–80.

36. Miralpeix E, Gonzalez-Comadran M, Sola I, Manau D, Carreras R, Checa MA. Efficacy of luteal phase support with vaginal progesterone in intrauterine insemination: a systematic review and meta-analysis. J Assist Reprod Genet 2014; 31:89–100.

37. Khosravi D, Taheripanah R, Taheripanah A, Monfared VT, Hosseini-Zijoud S. comparison of oral dydrogestrone with vaginal progesteronefor luteal support in IUI cycles: a randomized clinical trial. Iran J Reprod Med 2015;13:433–8.

38. Gopinath PM, Desai RR. Open label observational study to determine the success rate of first cycle of intrauterine insemination (IUI) involving luteal phase support with oral natural or synthe-tic progesterone. Int J Med Res Health Sci 2014;3: 933–6.

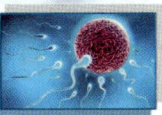

Sperm Banking: A Solution to all Problems

Anjali Malpani and Anirudhha Malpani

While recent advances in medical technology have dramatically improved the treatment options we can offer to the infertile man, the fact remains that many of these ART techniques are so expensive that they are out of the reach of most Indian couples. This is why the hoary treatment option of therapeutic insemination by donor (TID) is still a viable alternative for many couples. Also, a significant proportion of donor insemination treatment in this day and age is for single women and same sex couples.

How is it biologically possible to freeze and store sperm?

The process of cryopreservation of biological tissue involves: (1) brief exposure to molar concentrations of a mixture of a variety of cryoprotectant agents, such as glycerol, propanediol, dimethyl sulfoxide, or sucrose; (2) slow cooling to subzero temperatures; and (3) complete dehydration of the cell contents to prevent ice crystal formation that may damage the cells. Upon reaching the temperature of liquid nitrogen, –196°C, the sperm are placed in storage indefinitely, where they remain in a quiescent state of minimal molecular motion. All metabolic activity is suspended, which means they can be stored for years without being damaged. They regain their normal motility and fertilizing ability once they are thawed.

A new technique of freezing called *vitrification* avoids the damage caused by ice forming inside the cell by using a super high concentration of antifreeze (DMSO and ethylene glycol), and dropping the temperature so rapidly that the water inside the cell never becomes ice. It just instantaneously supercools into a solid with no ice crystal formation at all. However, this has still not been used widely for sperm freezing.

What is sperm banking?

Human sperm cryopreservation has become common in medical practice. The commonest indication is freezing sperm for donor insemination therapeutic insemination by donor (TID). Since it is dangerous to use fresh sperm for donor insemination because of the risk of transmitting infectious diseases such as AIDS and hepatitis B and hepatitis C, good clinics now use only frozen sperm for donor insemination after quarantining it and ensuring the donors are negative for infectious diseases.

What are the other uses for sperm banking?

While the major application of sperm banking today is for donor insemination, sperm banking is also useful in a number of other areas as well. Thus, we can store and freeze husband's sperm samples for treating the wife, and this is very useful in the following circumstances.

- When the husband has situational erectile dysfunction, so that he cannot produce a semen sample by masturbation at the appropriate time of an IUI or IVF cycle, storing a sample is very useful. This frozen sample can be used as a backup, in case the man cannot produce a sample at the required time. However, in many cases, because the man knows that a frozen sample is available, this helps to take the pressure off, so that many of them can produce a fresh sample with little difficulty!

- When the husband is away (working overseas or traveling), his frozen sample can be used to make pregnancy possible.

For men with cancers, sperm freezing offers them a chance of conserving their reproductive potential.

What are the advantages of using frozen sperm for donor insemination?

- No risk of STD and AIDS as the samples are quarantined and the donors are retested
- Around the clock availability; no scheduling bottle neck
- High quality product since it is tested before and after freezing
- Rh negative donors can be used for Rh negative women
- Physical traits of husband and donor can be matched.

Who are the donors?

The donors are healthy men between 20 to 40, from a sound background, and usually graduates. Those who are healthy, with no family history of illness are requested to provide a sperm sample for testing. This semen is analyzed, and accepted only if it has superior qualities: a count over 100 million per millimetre; and motility of 70 to 80%. Their blood is checked to make sure they are negative for infectious diseases. The physical traits of the donor are recorded, so that he can be matched with the husband's physical characters. The doctor matches the donor and the husband for height, build, hair colour, skin colour, eye colour, Rh factor and blood group. After the sample is frozen, it is quarantined; and the donor's blood re-tested after 6 months. Only when this second test is negative are the samples released for clinic use.

What are directed donors?

Sometimes couples wish to use a friend or relative as donor. However, there are dangers in doing so. Overtime, the donor's psychological make-up as well as the relationship with the donor may change. This could create social and legal problems. Furthermore, you will become dependent upon the donor's discretion to keep the insemination a secret. This is why using a known donor is not usually a good idea–however tempting this may seem.

How is the sperm frozen and stored in a sperm bank?

After liquefaction, the semen sample is mixed with an equal quantity of the cryoprotectant medium (a chemical which prevents the sperm from being damaged even at very low temperatures) and is loaded into plastic vials or straws. These are uniquely coded and sealed; and then placed in steel tubs of liquid nitrogen where they are frozen to $-196°C$. One day later, one straw is removed and thawed to see how the sperms survived the cold (cryosurvival). Only samples which contain at least 25 to 40 million motile sperm are accepted.

How is donor insemination treatment performed?

The couple signs a consent form for TID after appropriate counseling. You should perform the basic tests to check the wife's fertility,

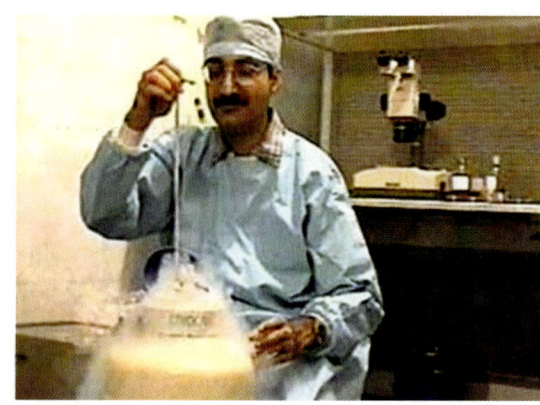

Fig. 11.1: Sperm being frozen in liquid nitrogen.

including a HSG to confirm tubal patency. She may be treated with fertility drugs for superovulation to improve pregnancy rates. Ovulation can be tracked by using ovulation test kits (for checking the LH surge) or doing vaginal ultrasound scans from the 11th day of the cycle. When ovulation occurs, the insemination is performed. A straw or vial of the appropriate donor is picked out from the liquid nitrogen and thawed. Please be very careful when handling liquid nitrogen. If it spills on your skin, it can cause a cold burn. The sample is thawed by simply leaving the straw at room temperature for 5 minutes. The sample is expelled into a sterile vial; and checked under the microscope to see that the sperm are actively motile. Under sterile conditions, the donor sperm is injected through a plastic catheter into the cervix.

How long can the sperm be frozen?
Since all metabolic activity is suspended at – 196, the sperm can theoretically be cryopreserved for ever.

Does sperm freezing cause an abnormal child?
This is a major concern patients have; and they can be reassured that the pregnancy is just like a normal pregnancy–with the same risks of miscarriage and birth defects as any other.

Should the child be told about TID?
With TID strict confidentiality is maintained, and the identities of the patients and donors are kept secret. Historically, parents have kept TID a secret from the child and from friends and relatives. Unlike adoption, TID is not obvious to those who know the infertile couple. It is entirely up to the parents to tell the child the circumstances of his or her birth and most Indian doctors advice against it. However, there is always the burden of secrecy which the parents have to bear for the rest of their life.

What about finding the donor's identity in the future?
Some countries like the UK have passed laws which allow the child to find out the identity of the donor once the child becomes 18. This has been done to protect the child's right to know, though it is still unclear whether this serves a useful purpose. As a result of this law, it is becoming increasingly difficult to recruit sperm donors in the UK.

How can sperm samples be shipped?
It is possible to transport frozen sperm samples around the world, as long as the cold chain is maintained. This is best done by transporting them in special dry shippers, whose walls are charged with nitrogen vapor which keeps the samples at −40°C. There is no risk of the liquid nitrogen spilling when these shippers are used.

How should couples be counseled for donor insemination?
Before a couple choose TID as a treatment, they must remember the taxing ethical, emotional and psychological repercussions it has for both of them. The husband may feel threatened, isolated, inferior, insecure and jealous. He may wonder whether he will be able to play father to 'another man's child'. In fact, with the advent of microinjection, coming to terms with TID has become even more difficult, since many men are forced to resort to TID rather than use microinjection with their own sperm purely for financial reasons.

The woman may be resentful that she has to undergo treatment and turmoil for something that is not actually her 'fault'. She may also worry about bearing the baby of a total stranger; and will often have no support as this is something which she may not be able to share with anyone–even her own mother.

Couples undergoing TID often undergo psychologic reactions which can be difficult to cope with. The sense of isolation is even more than with other forms of infertility, since most couples do not tell anyone they are undergoing AID—so that they miss the social support and sympathy which other infertile patients receive. The stress can be tremendous because the sperms of another man are being inseminated into the wife, and both partners experience many conflicting emotions. The involvement of a completely unknown third party as a sperm donor can make coping with the pregnancy especially difficult. Fantasies and nightmares may occur about the unknown donor—and there are also concerns as to whether the child will be normal and what the child will look like. Many men also experience sexual impotency at this time, but this is only temporary.

What are the ethical and legal issues with sperm and embryo banking?

Men whose sperm are to be frozen should give their informed consent before the cryopreservation. The elements of an appropriate consent form should include a description of the procedures involved in freezing and thawing, the risks (a mechanical failure of a catastrophic event leading to the loss of the frozen sperm, failure of the sperm to survive freezing and thawing) and benefits (preservation of fertility), alternatives (disposal of the sperm before thawing), and disposition of the frozen sperm in the case of the death of the person from whom the tissue was obtained, divorce or dissolution of a partnership in the case of embryos, nonpayment of storage fees, and loss of contact with the person. Many countries now have laws which regulate these procedures.

What are the quality control issues in sperm banking?

Sperm banks are faced with the specter of expanding inventories and potential cross-contamination of specimens that could be infected with viruses and are stored in communal liquid nitrogen tanks. Long-term storage of sperm poses a logistic problem for a fertility clinic, for potentially infected samples should be maintained in separate tanks to avoid cross-contamination. Among the alternatives available in such circumstances are: on-site storage in nitrogen vapor or off-site storage at facilities specializing in maintaining large inventories of potentially infectious samples. It is a good idea to use an electronic database to maintain the inventory of the sperm, and there are many software programs available which do this well.

SUGGESTED READING

1. Johnson MD, Cooper AR, Jungheim ES, Lanzendorf SE, Odem RR, Ratts VS. Sperm banking for fertility preservation: a 20-year experience. Eur J Obstet Gynecol Reprod Biol. 2013;170(1): 177–82.

2. Yogev L, Kleiman SE, Shabtai E, Botchan A, Paz G, Hauser R, Lehavi O, Yavetz H, Gamzu R. Long-term cryostorage of sperm in a human sperm bank does not damage progressive motility concentration. Hum Reprod 2010;25(5):1097–103.

3. Dan Gong, Yu-Lin Liu, Zhong Zheng, Yi-Fei Tian, and Zheng Li. An overview on ethical issues about sperm donation. Asian J Androl 2009;11(6): 645–52.

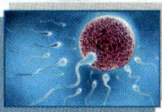

12

Medicolegal Aspect of IUI

Manish Machave

'Hope' is the thing with feathers–That perches in the soul–
And sings the tune without the words–And never stops-at all

Emily Dickinson

INTRODUCTION

It is estimated that 15% of couples around the world are infertile. This implies that infertility is one of the highly prevalent medical problems. The magnitude of the infertility problem also has enormous social implications. Besides the fact that every couple has the right to have a child, in India infertility widely carries with it a social stigma. In the Indian social context specially, children are also a kind of old age insurance.

The rationale behind artificial insemination is increasing the gamete density at the site of fertilization. Since many centuries different pioneers contributed to the history of artificial insemination, not only in humans but even more pronounced in farm animals. The primary reason for using this technique in farm animals was to speed up the rate of genetic improvement by increasing the productivity of food producing animals. This was accomplished by improving the selection differential wherein one highly selected male is mated with thousands of females. The AID industry was born.

For humans the situation is different: artificial insemination was originally developed to help couples to conceive in case of severe male factor subfertility of a physical or psychological nature. Nowadays artificial insemination with homologous semen is most commonly used for unexplained and mild male factor subfertility. In the previous century donor insemination was mainly used for male infertility due to azoospermia or very low sperm count and for inherited genetic diseases linked to the Y-chromosome. Nowadays donor insemination is more commonly used in women with no male partner (lesbians or single women).

HISTORY OF IUI

Henry IV (1425–1474), **King of Castile**, married Princess Juana. The queen got pregnant after 6 long years of marriage and delivered a daughter. Henry IV was said to be impotent and historians claim that he might be the one who first tried artificial insemination. The possibility of artificial insemination was launched. Later on it was claimed that the princess was not the daughter of the king.

LANDMARKS IN IUI

1677 • Van Leeuwenhoek Antoni
First picture of sperm cells

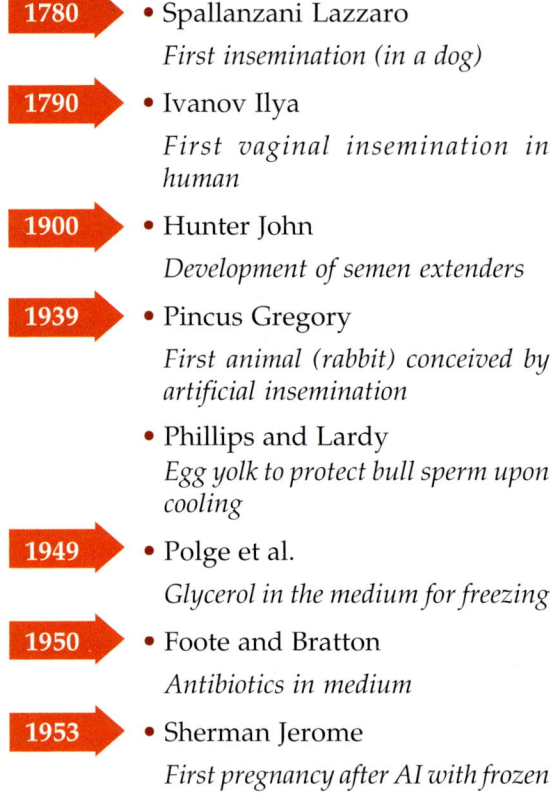

1780
- Spallanzani Lazzaro

  First insemination (in a dog)

1790
- Ivanov Ilya

  First vaginal insemination in human

1900
- Hunter John

  Development of semen extenders

1939
- Pincus Gregory

  First animal (rabbit) conceived by artificial insemination

- Phillips and Lardy

  Egg yolk to protect bull sperm upon cooling

1949
- Polge et al.

  Glycerol in the medium for freezing

1950
- Foote and Bratton

  Antibiotics in medium

1953
- Sherman Jerome

  First pregnancy after AI with frozen sperm

1978
- Steptoe and Edwards

  First IVF birth—refinement of semen processing techniques Medicolegal Aspects of IUI

Artificial insemination faced the fire when discussions first erupted in USA around 1909. It was questioned as it was thought to defy moral and religious grounds. Europe joined to see this as a technique as a vice, rather than seeing it is a technique which could gift infertile couples with children. Artificial insemination of donor semen (AID) was widely objected as it was said to promote vice of masturbation alone with potential encouragement of eugenic government policies.

Nevertheless, the demand for donor sperm increased tremendously. After the first successful pregnancy from frozen sperm, reported in 1953, the development of a thriving sperm-bank industry starting in the 1970s and the commercialization of AID became unavoidable. As the number of AID increased, the chances of sexually transmitted diseases also raised, which brought in some of the regulations making it mandatory to screen the semen to be used for insemination.

One more possibility with AID was: in view of keeping confidentiality, multiple usage of donor semen might lead to fusion with biologically connected female's ovum. So, to prevent such mishap, some of the governments brought in some regulations to limit the times a donor semen can be used or limit the number of children conceived with usage of the particular donor semen.

We in India are governed basically by two sets of regulations in this aspect. The National Guidelines for Accreditation, Supervision and Regulation of ART Clinics in India, by the Indian Council of Medical Research (ICMR) and the National Academy of Medical Sciences, India, 2005 and The Assisted Reproductive Technology (Regulation) Rules, 2010.

LEGAL ASPECTS RELATED TO IUI

Registration of Clinic

A new ART clinic needs to obtain a temporary registration. This registration needs to be confirmed by obtaining accreditation (permanent registration) from the center or State's appropriate accreditation authority within next two years of temporary registration. *Every seven years, this registration needs to be renewed.*

Existing ART clinic needs to obtain temporary registration within six months of receiving notification from accreditation authority, after which a permanent registration needs to be obtained within next two years.

Process of Accreditation

A State Accreditation Authority will be set-up by the State Governments through its Department of Health and/or Family Welfare to oversee all policy matters relating to accreditation, supervision and regulation of ART clinics in the states in accordance with the National Guidelines.

The State Government may also set-up *appropriate authorities* for implementation of the guidelines for the whole or a part of State having regard to the number of the ART clinics and delegate powers to impose a fine or a penalty on the center/clinic.

In addition to the above, the Ministry of Health and Family Welfare, Govternment of India, will set-up a *National Advisory Committee* which will advise the Central Government on policy matters relating to regulation of ART Clinics.

TYPES OF INFERTILITY CLINICS

Primary Level 1

- Preliminary investigations
- Diagnosis of infertility
- *Do not require handling of sperm, egg, embryo outside the body*
- Consulting room, general hospital
- Responsibilities—**Counseling/history/ examination/treatment.**

Secondary Level 2

- Require registration under ART act
- Facilities of AIH/AID/IUI
- *Except oocytes handled outside the body*
- Responsibilities—**SFT/TVS/hysteroscopy/ laparoscopy**
- **Except**—Provision for oocyte pick-up.

Tertiary Level 3

- Require registration under the act
- All except research on the human embryos
- In case all facilities not available-should HV access to such at other app accreditated **ART Bank or Lab**
- Responsibilities—**Cryopreservation of gametes and embryos.**

ETHICS COMMITTEE

Each ART clinic of levels 1B, 2 and 3 must have its own Ethics Committee constituted

according to ICMR guidelines, comprising reputed ART practitioners, scientists who are knowledgeable in developmental biology or in clinical embryology, a social scientist, a member of the judiciary and a person who are well-versed in comparative theology.

CONSENTS FOR IUI (ART BILL, ICMR GUIDELINES)

Consent for Artificial Insemination or Intra-uterine Insemination with Husband's Semen/ Sperm (See Rule 15.1).

_____ and _____ ____, being husband and wife and both of legal age, authorize Dr._____ to inseminate the wife artificially or intrauterine with the semen/ sperm of the husband for achieving conception.

We understand that even though the insemination may be repeated as often as recommended by the doctor, there is no guarantee or assurance that pregnancy or a live birth will result.

We have also been told that the outcome of pregnancy may not be the same as those of the general pregnant population, e.g. in respect of abortion, multiple pregnancies, anomalies or complications of pregnancy or delivery.

The procedure carried out does not ensure a positive result, nor does it guarantee a mentally and physically normal child. This consent holds good for all the cycles performed at the clinic.

Endorsement by the ART Clinic

I / we have personally explained to _____ and _____ the details and implications of his/her/their signing this consent/ approval form, and made sure to the extent humanly possible that he/she/they understand these details and implications.

Name, address and signature of the witness from the clinic

Signed: _____ (Husband)

_____(Wife)

_____
Name and signature of the Doctor

_____

_____
Name and address of the ART clinic

Dated:

FORM-F Consent for Artificial Insemination or Intrauterine Insemination with Donor Semen (See Rule 15.1)

We,_____and _____,
being husband and wife and both of legal age, authorize Dr._____ to inseminate the wife
artificially or intrauterine with the semen/ sperm of
a donor (ARTb bank's no._____; obtained
from _____ART bank with valid registration
no_____) for achieving conception.

We understand that even though the insemination
may be repeated as often as recommended by the
doctor, there is no guarantee or assurance that
pregnancy or a live birth will result.

We have also been told that the outcome of pregnancy
may not be the same as those of the general pregnant
population, e.g. in respect of abortion, multiple
pregnancies, anomalies or complications of pregnancy
or delivery.

We declare that we shall not attempt to find out the
identity of the donor.

I, the husband, also declare that should my wife
bear any child or children as a result of such
insemination(s), such child or children shall be as my
own and shall be my legal heir(s).

The procedure carried out does not ensure a positive
result, nor does it guarantee a mentally and physically
normal body. This consent holds good for all the
cycles performed at the clinic.

Endorsement by the ART Clinic

I /we have personally explained to _____
and _____ the details and implications
of his/her/their signing this consent/approval form,
and made sure to the extent humanly possible that
he/she/they understand these details and implications.

Name, address and signature of the witness from the
clinic
Signed: _____ (Husband)

            _____(Wife)

_____
Name and signature of the Doctor

_____

_____
Name and address of the ART clinic
Dated:
_____
Note: An appropriate modification of this form may
be used for artificial insemination or intrauterine
insemination of a single woman with donor semen.

HOW TO PROCURE SPERMS FOR AID?

The collection, screening and storage of
semen; and provision of oocyte donor and
surrogates, shall be done by an *ART bank
registered as an independent entity under the
provisions of this Act. An ART bank shall operate
independently of any assisted reproductive
technology clinic.*

Semen from males between twenty-one
years of age and forty-five years of age, both
inclusive, examine the donors for such
diseases, sexually transmitted or otherwise,
as may be prescribed, and all other commu-
nicable diseases which may endanger the
health of the parents, or any one of them,
surrogate or child. All ART banks shall cryo-
preserve sperm donations for a quarantine
period of at least six months before being used
and, at the expiry of such period.

An ART bank may advertise for gamete
donors and surrogates, who may be compen-
sated financially by the bank. An ART bank
shall not supply the sperm of a single donor
for use more than seventy-five times. One
sample of semen supplied by an ART bank
shall be used by the assisted reproductive
technology clinic only once on only one
recipient.

An assisted reproductive technology clinic
*shall never mix semen from two individuals before
use.* No ART clinic shall obtain or use sperm
or oocyte donated by relative or known friend
of either of the parties seeking ART treatment
or procedures.

An ART bank may, for such appropriate
fee as may be prescribed, store any semen
obtained from a donor for the exclusive use
of the wife or partner of the donor.

Records of such are to be maintained for a
period of 10 years and then sent to ICMR/
ART DATBASE.

CONFIDENTIALITY

Information in respect of a sperm or oocyte
donor or a surrogate, including the name,
identity and address of such donor or

surrogate shall be kept confidential. Personal information-personal identification will not be released without the prior informed consent of the genetic parent or parents or surrogate mother.

WHEN WITHELD INFORMATION MAY BE DISCLOSED

In pursuance of an order or decree of a court of competent jurisdiction.

A child may, upon reaching the age of 18, ask for any information, excluding personal relating to the donor or surrogate mother.

Legal guardian, excluding personal, for welfare of the child.

Personal identification of the genetic parent or parents or surrogate mother may be released only in cases of life-threatening medical conditions which require physical testing or samples of the genetic parent or parents or surrogate mother.

STATUS OF CHILD BORN OUT OF AID

In case of a married couple and insemination is done with due consent the child born shall have all legal rights as a legitimate child born through sexual intercourse.

In case of unmarried couple and insemination is done with due consent the child born shall have all legal rights and shall be the legitimate child of both parties.

In case of single man/woman and insemination is done with due consent the child born shall have all legal rights and shall be the legitimate child of the single man/woman.

In case there is divorce/separation of couple after ART but before birth, the child born shall be the legitimate child of couple.

A child born to a woman artificially inseminated with the stored sperm of her dead husband shall be considered as the legitimate child of the couple.

BIRTH CERTIFICATE AND CITIZENSHIP

The birth certificate of a child born through the use of assisted reproductive technology shall contain the name or names of the parent or parents, as the case may be, who sought such use.

If a foreigner or a foreign couple seeks sperm or egg donation, or surrogacy, in India, and a child is born as a consequence, the child, even though born in India, shall not be an Indian citizen.

Grey Areas in the Present Legislation

Redefining 'legitimacy': The guidelines recommend going beyond the outdated Indian Evidence Act, 1872, that limits legitimacy of a child born to only within 280 days after dissolution of marriage (by death or divorce): 'The law needs to take note of the scientific advancements since that time. Thus a child born to a woman artificially inseminated with the stored sperms of her deceased husband must be considered to be a legitimate child notwithstanding the existing law of presumptions under our evidence act. The law needs to move along with medical advancements and suitably amended so that it does not give rise to dilemma or unwarranted harsh situations.'

However, in the main, as a document that should ideally lay down guiding principles for research and practice related to ARTs, the guidelines fall short.

Informed consent not ensured: The crucial issue of informed consent is dealt with rather summarily and in vague terms: 'More particularly, the clinic must make sure that patients are well-informed about the treatment being offered to them, the reasons of suggesting a particular form of treatment, and alternative therapies available if any.' Chapter 3, dealing with ethical and legal considerations, talks only about written consent (3.2.5), but fails to make informed consent mandatory. In fact, the nine sample consent forms in Chapter 4 seem designed more to insure the clinic and medical personnel from legal action, rather than to protect the rights of the individuals accessing ARTs. While conducting clinical trials or offering newer and experimental procedures, it should be ensured that the person is provided adequate and comprehensible information. Information about the potential risks and benefits should be provided verbally as well as in written form in simple, easily understandable language with minimum use of technical jargon. Written information should be provided in the regional language whenever necessary, even for newer, potentially complicated procedures.

Rigid notions of family: In what at first reading might appear to be a progressive move, the guidelines recommend that there be no bar to the use of ART by a single woman who wishes to have a child, and no ART clinic may refuse to offer its services to her. Interestingly, the entire section (3.16.4) has been deleted in the corrigendum.

What pressures or re-thinking led to this last minute deletion?

In general, ARTs should be made available to any consenting adults who desire to have a child using these technological innovations. Neither the marital status of the persons (married, unmarried, single, divorced) nor their sexual orientation (heterosexual, homosexual or bisexual) should be used as a decision-making criterion. Changing social trends the world over should be kept in mind while setting up ethical guidelines, and accordingly the words 'husband' and 'wife' must be substituted by 'male partner' and 'female partner'.

The guidelines state that the clinic and the couple shall have the right to have the fullest possible information from the semen bank about the donor, such as height, weight, skin colour, educational qualification, profession, and family background. This reinforces the regressive notion that intelligence is strictly associated with these criteria.

Legal, sociocultural and religious considerations surrounding artificial donor insemination.

Many countries are still in view of having heterosexual couple as a base for a family. There have been sociocultural resistance in many countries with regards to aloowing semen donation for single mothers of homosexual females. Few more potential question would be: how and what to tell those children born out of AID about their parent if the donor anonymous. In case of non-anonymous donors, whether to tell children and if yes, when and how to tell about their biological parents. There have been many more ethical and moral such questions including usage of brother's or father's semen. Whether or not to pay the donors and sexing of sperm by DNA quantification using flow cytometry instrumentation became a point of discussion.

CONCLUSION

While the guidelines attempt to incorporate some issues related to social justice and gender inequality, they still fall short on many fronts. In this era of rapidly advancing technologies, ethical guidelines need to have proper safeguards making it a balanced environment for both providers and users of those particular techniques. The guidelines should also keep in mind the unequal gender balance and ensure that the rights of women users of these technologies are not compromised in any manner.

The very title 'National guidelines for accreditation, supervision and regulation of ART clinics in India' makes it clear that the ICMR, the apex body in India for the formulation, coordination, and promotion of biomedical research, has limited itself to creating red tape on the running of clinics. It is critical of us to envision future trends and create an ethical infrastructure for biomedical research, especially in this era of newer techniques for human reproduction that could expand the horizons of humanity. This role, it seems, is not one that the ICMR is ready to play.

BIBLIOGRAPHY

1. Belonoschkin B. The science of reproduction and its traditions. Int J Fertil 1956;1:215–24.

2. Bensdorp AJ, Cohlen BJ, Heineman MJ, van Dekerckhove P. Intra-uterine insemination for male subfertility. Cochrane Database Syst Rev 2007;4(CD000360).

3. Cohlen BJ. Should we continue performing intra-uterine inseminations in the year 2004? Gynecol Obstet Invest 2005;59:3–13.

4. Cohlen B, Ombelet W. Intra-Uterine Insemination: Evidence-Based Guidelines for Daily Practice. Boca Raton, US: CRC Press, Taylor & Francis Group; 2014.

5. ESHRE Capri Workshop Group. Intrauterine insemination. Hum Reprod Update 2009;15:265–77.

6. Kremer J. The significance of Antoni van Leeuwenhoek for the early development of Andrology. Andrologia 1979;11:234–49.

7. Laxmi Murthy, Vani Subramanian ICMR guidelines on Assisted Reproductive Technology: lacking in vision, wrapped in red tape DOI: https://doi.org/10.20529/IJME.2007.049.

8. Perry EJ. The Artificial Insemination of Farm Animals. 4th ed. New Brunswick, New York: Rutgers University Press 1968.

9. Phillips EJ, Lardy HA. A yolk-buffer pabulum for the preservation of bull semen. J Dairy Sci. 1940; 23:399–404.

10. Stoughton RH. Artificial human insemination. Nature 1948;13:790.

11. van Leeuwenhoek A. De natis è semine genital animalculis. Vol. 12. R. Soc. (Lond.) Philos Trans 1678;1040–3.

Index